ASSISTED SUICIDE

Medical Ethics

David H. Smith and Robert M. Veatch, *Editors*

VOLUME 25 IN THE SERIES

Assisted Suicide

FINDING COMMON GROUND

Edited by

LOIS SNYDER

AND

ARTHUR L. CAPLAN

INDIANA UNIVERSITY PRESS

Bloomington and
Indianapolis

This book is a publication of
Indiana University Press
601 North Morton Street
Bloomington, Indiana 47404-3797 USA
http://iupress.indiana.edu

Telephone orders   800-842-6796
Fax orders   812-855-7931
Orders by e-mail   iuporder@indiana.edu

The paper used in this publication meets the minimum requirements of American National Standard for Information Sciences—Permanence of Paper for
Printed Library Materials, ANSI Z39.48-1984.

Manufactured in the United States of America

Library of Congress Cataloging-in-Publication Data

Assisted suicide : finding common ground / edited by Lois Snyder and
Arthur L. Caplan.
p.   cm. — (Medical ethics series)
Includes bibliographical references and index.
ISBN 0-253-33977-4
1. Assisted suicide. I. Snyder, Lois, date. II. Caplan, Arthur L. III. Series.
R726 .A855 2002
174′.24—dc21
2001001108

1 2 3 4 5   07 06 05 04 03 02

To

Hannah and Zach

CONTENTS

ACKNOWLEDGMENTS

Grant Support: The editors and the Assisted Suicide Consensus Panel wish to thank the Walter and Elise Haas Fund for support of the development of the papers in the Finding Common Ground Project series and generous support of the development of this book. We also would like to thank the Wallace Alexander Gerbode Foundation for support of the project.

Members of the Assisted Suicide Consensus Panel convened by the University of Pennsylvania Center for Bioethics (1997–2000) were: Lois Snyder, J.D. (University of Pennsylvania, Philadelphia, Pa.), *Project Director;* Arthur L. Caplan, Ph.D. (University of Pennsylvania, Philadelphia, Pa.), *Chair;* David A. Asch, M.D., M.B.A. (University of Pennsylvania, Philadelphia, Pa.); Rev. Ralph Ciampa (University of Pennsylvania, Philadelphia, Pa.); Kathy Faber-Langendoen, M.D. (SUNY Health Sciences Center, Syracuse, N.Y.); Joseph J. Fins, M.D. (Weill Medical College of Cornell University, New York, N.Y.); John Hansen-Flaschen, M.D. (University of Pennsylvania, Philadelphia, Pa.); Barbara Coombs Lee, P.A., F.N.P., J.D. (Compassion in Dying Federation, Portland, Ore.); Franklin G. Miller, Ph.D. (University of Virginia, Charlottesville, Va.); Sally J. Nunn, R.N. (University of Pennsylvania, Philadelphia, Pa.); David Orentlicher, M.D., J.D. (Indiana University School of Law, Indianapolis, Ind.); Timothy E. Quill, M.D. (The Genessee Hospital, Rochester, N.Y.); Elliott J. Rosen, Ed.D. (Family Institute of Westchester, Scarsdale, N.Y.); and James A. Tulsky, M.D. (Durham Veterans Affairs Medical Center and Duke University Medical Center, Durham, N.C.).

Journal Acknowledgments and Panel Member Dissents:
Prior versions of the Assisted Suicide Consensus Panel publications appeared as:

L. Snyder and A. L. Caplan, for the University of Pennsylvania Center for Bioethics Assisted Suicide Consensus Panel, "Assisted Suicide: Finding Common Ground," *Annals of Internal Medicine* 132 (2000): 468–469.

F. G. Miller, J. J. Fins, and L. Snyder for the University of Pennsylvania Center for Bioethics Assisted Suicide Consensus Panel, "Assisted Suicide Compared with Refusal of Treatment: A Valid Distinction?" *Annals of Internal Medicine* 132 (2000): 470–475. Barbara Coombs Lee, David Orentlicher, and Timothy Quill dissented from the paper.

A. L. Caplan, L. Snyder, and K. Faber-Langendoen for the University of Pennsylvania Center for Bioethics Assisted Suicide Consensus Panel, "The Role of Guidelines in the Practice of Physician-Assisted Suicide," *Annals of Internal Medicine* 132 (2000): 476–481.

K. Faber-Langendoen and J. H. Karlawish for the University of Pennsylvania Center for Bioethics Assisted Suicide Consensus Panel, "Should Assisted Suicide Be Only Physician Assisted?" *Annals of Internal Medicine* 132 (2000): 482–487. Barbara Coombs Lee, Timothy Quill, and Lois Snyder dissented from the paper.

T. E. Quill, B.C. Lee, and S. Nunn for the University of Pennsylvania Center for Bioethics Assisted Suicide Consensus Panel, "Palliative Treatments of Last Resort: Choosing the Least Harmful Alternative," *Annals of Internal Medicine* 132 (2000): 488–493. Joseph Fins dissented from the paper.

J. A. Tulsky, R. Ciampa, and E. J. Rosen for the University of Pennsylvania Center for Bioethics Assisted Suicide Consensus Panel, "Responding to Legal Requests for Physician-Assisted Suicide," *Annals of Internal Medicine* 132 (2000): 494–499.
Copyright 2000 by *Annals of Internal Medicine*. All rights reserved. Used with permission.

D. Orentlicher and L. Snyder for the University of Pennsylvania Center for Bioethics Assisted Suicide Consensus Panel, "Can Assisted Suicide Be Regulated?" *Journal of Clinical Ethics* 11, no. 4 (2001): 358–366. Joseph Fins, Barbara Coombs Lee, and Franklin Miller dissented from the paper. Copyright 2001 by *The Journal of Clinical Ethics*. All rights reserved. Used with permission. www.clinicalethics.com

ASSISTED SUICIDE

INTRODUCTION

LOIS SNYDER, J.D., AND ARTHUR L. CAPLAN, PH.D.

Assisted Suicide: Finding Common Ground

IT IS HERE. Support it. Oppose it. Be neutral. But do not ignore it. Physician-assisted suicide is no longer a theoretical issue just for academic debate.

The United States Supreme Court has ruled that there is no constitutional right to assisted suicide.[1] Most states explicitly criminalize it. But they can also allow it, and Oregon has chosen to legalize physician-assisted suicide in certain circumstances under detailed procedures.[2] Articles in the *New England Journal of Medicine* in February 1999 and February 2000 describe the implementation of the law in years one and two, when twenty-three and thirty-three people, respectively, were reported as having received prescriptions for lethal medications from physicians under the Oregon law.[3]

Some view the ability to control the manner and timing of death in this way as a right. Inadequacies in end-of-life care continue to make legalization an appealing option, or at least an option many view as worth having, and well-organized efforts to legalize physician-assisted suicide continue. Consideration of the Pain Relief Promotion Act of 1999 and other bills in Congress has kept physician-assisted suicide on the national policy and legislative agenda.

Proponents and opponents will view the initial Oregon experience differently. Those in favor will say the law is working well, that the small numbers indicate that the floodgates have not, in fact, been opened, and that no abuses have occurred. Those opposed will suspect underreporting as in the Netherlands and will highlight that the individuals who were ending their lives were not reported to have been in pain or suffering, which were supposed to be the most compelling reasons for supporting the practice (this finding was more prominent in the first-year report, based on interviews with physicians about why individuals said they were requesting physician-assisted suicide; the second-year information included interviews with physicians and with family members).[4]

In early 1997, anticipating that it would become legal—as it did in Oregon at the end of that year—we organized a project at the University of Pennsylvania's Center for Bioethics to convene a national panel of experts on the subject of assisted suicide. The panel membership was multidisciplinary—with representatives from medicine, nursing, psychology, hospice, patient advocacy, law, philosophy, the clergy, and bioethics. It was deliberately composed of individuals with diverse viewpoints on assisted suicide, those for and against. Our goal was not to argue the pros or cons. Instead, starting from the assumption that legalization was coming, we sought to find common ground in examining how to guide practices and determine safeguards that would keep assisted suicide voluntary, regulated, and an option of last resort.

Did we avoid the "real" issue by not deciding the morality of assisted suicide? That is certainly an important question. But it is not the only question, and it is not today the urgent question. Assisted suicide, particularly physician-assisted suicide, is popularly supported and is now going on legally. These facts do not make it "right," but, clearly, some guidance about its practice is needed. Groups in the past who have come together to try to write guidelines have failed when the discussion shifted from how to do so, back to whether to do so. In the process, important policy considerations about how to keep physician-assisted suicide rare, alternatives to the practice, the implications for the patient-physician relationship, who should write guidelines, and how to regulate it were not getting addressed.

The Assisted Suicide Consensus Panel of the Finding Common Ground Project debated a number of questions, often loudly: What is assisted suicide? Is physician-assisted suicide different from refusal of treatment? Are there alternatives to assisted suicide? How useful are currently available guidelines for physician-assisted suicide? Who should have access to what? Does assisted suicide necessarily mean physician-assisted suicide? Can it be effectively and meaningfully regulated? How should physicians respond to requests for assisted suicide? Results of the panel's deliberations and consensus process included papers published in medical and ethics journals.[5] Panel members did not agree on everything. Given the differing points of view, total agreement was not expected. But we did find much and important, if not always rock-hard, common ground.

This book offers expanded versions of the consensus papers and additional chapters, background material, and food for thought. Context is provided by Oregon experts on the early years of the implementation of that state's physician-assisted suicide law and the implications for end-of-life care in Oregon. Then, Chapter 2, "Assisted Suicide and Refusal of Treatment: Valid Distinction or Distinction without a Difference?," starts the policy debate at the beginning, with an examination of definitions and first principles. The continuing debate often confuses how physician-assisted suicide is like or not like the refusal of life-sustaining treatment. But ethics and policy considerations can turn on whether or not there is a valid distinction between assisted suicide and the withdrawal/withholding of treatment. This chapter examines leading arguments for and against recognizing a fundamental distinction, using three cases: an assisted suicide by ingestion of prescribed barbiturates, a withdrawal of artificial nutrition and hydration, and a decision to stop eating and drinking. In particular, arguments about causation, physician intention, and bodily integrity are analyzed. On theoretical and practical grounds, it is argued that there is a valid distinction between assisted suicide and refusal of treatment.

In Chapter 3, "The Role of Guidelines in the Practice of Physician-Assisted Suicide," the moral import of attempting to formulate guidelines; the utility of guidelines on the actual practice of doctors, health care providers, patients or families; and whether any set of guidelines can really protect against harm or abuse are considered. What has been the experience of efforts to implement physician-assisted suicide using consensus guidelines? What goals do guidelines serve? Who should formulate them? What barriers are there to the creation and implementation of guidelines? And, fundamentally, is dying a process that is amenable to direction under guidelines by physicians, departments of health, blue-ribbon panels, or other regulatory bodies? Here a concern is that the debate about guidelines to regulate the practice of physician-assisted suicide has been shaped more by overall attitudes about the desirability or undesirability of legalization than by any particular set of guidelines and their merit. This has served to narrow the debate. In addition, guidelines have mostly been seen as rules for doctors, often disconnected from patient and family views of suffering and death and from religious and spiritual frameworks.

Next, in Chapter 4 the question is posed, "Ought Assisted Suicide Be Only *Physician* Assisted?" The assumption inherent in many discussions in the media, in courts, in legislatures, at dinner tables, and in other settings—that assistance with suicide generally means physician-assisted suicide—is questioned. This chapter seeks to define both the necessity and the limits of the physician's role in assisted suicide. It concludes that assisted suicide requires physician involvement, but physicians' limited competence in performing the full range of tasks, the competencies of other professions, and the possibility that other professions could expand their authority in this area indicate that *physician*-assisted suicide is too narrow a construct.

Chapter 5, "Can Assisted Suicide Be Regulated?," takes a hard look at important questions about how possible it is to regulate a legal right to assisted suicide. Assuming that there are times when assisted suicide is morally acceptable in theory, it addresses whether a right to assisted suicide that is morally safe can be implemented in practice. That is, can regulations for assisted suicide that will truly prevent serious abuse be designed? Or are the difficulties with regulation so severe that it is preferable for patients to rely on the alternatives to suicide that are currently permitted (e.g., terminal sedation and/or the refusal of food and water)? Can useful analogies be made to regulation in other contexts?

"Palliative Treatments of Last Resort: Choosing the Least Harmful Alternative," Chapter 6, looks at how physicians, nurses, patients, families, and loved ones still can face clinically, ethically, morally, and legally challenging decisions throughout the dying process even when palliative care is effective. This is especially so for the terminally ill patient who, in the face of complex, difficult-to-treat suffering, is ready to die and requests assistance from health care providers. Although physician-assisted suicide has received the most attention as a potential last resort, decisions are made more commonly regarding accelerating opioids for pain, forgoing life-sustaining therapy, voluntarily stopping eating and drinking, and terminal sedation, in an attempt to respond to unacceptable terminal suffering. The moral distinctions between these practices are critical to some and relatively inconsequential to others. This chapter illustrates, with summaries of real clinical cases, how each of these practices might be a response to patients in particular clinical circumstances, keeping in focus the patient's values, as well as those of families, other loved ones, and health care providers. It describes the challenge of finding the least harmful solution to the patient's dilemma, without abandoning the patient to unacceptable suffering or leaving him or her to act in a more deleterious way alone. It maintains that any intervention that is likely to hasten death should be considered only as a last resort, when life has become intolerable to the patient in the face of unrestrained efforts to relieve suffering, and that physician-assisted suicide should be kept exceedingly rare.

In Chapter 7, "Responding to Legal Requests for Physician-Assisted

Suicide," how the physician responds to requests in an era of legalization is examined. When legal, physician-assisted suicide becomes one of the many options to be freely considered for terminally ill patients with extreme suffering, and some patients will view it as a right to expect on demand. This chapter considers the ethical implications of disclosing to patients assisted suicide as an option of last resort. Physicians, however, even when practicing in jurisdictions that allow it, should not encourage patients to hasten death. Further, without abandoning the model, it is suggested that strict informed consent does not fully address patients' needs at this time. Physicians must also focus on broader biopsychosocial concerns and, through empathic listening and emotional support, help the patient identify solutions. A context and vocabulary for physicians when responding to requests for assisted suicide are provided. Physicians should clarify the request, explore and address the patient's concerns, achieve a shared understanding of the goals of treatment, search for less harmful alternatives, express to the patient what they are willing to do, discuss the relevant legal issues, and share their decision making with colleagues.

"Lesson from the Dying," Chapter 8, then brings some (purposely uncomfortable) closure, as death and dying and suicide and assisted suicide are viewed in personal, and professional, perspective.

An annotated bibliography on assisted suicide follows, along with appendices on the Oregon Death with Dignity Act and the texts of the 1997 U.S. Supreme Court decisions on the topic, *Washington et al. v. Glucksberg et al.* and *Vacco, Attorney General of New York, et al. v. Quill et al.*

All in all, we think that this volume will contribute to advancing the policy dialogue and assist those who will be dealing with these issues in practice. Taken together, these chapters form a framework for what assisted suicide, particularly physician-assisted suicide, is, and how its legalized practice might be guided. Some commentators may fault this work for not starting with a uniformity of opinion on its legalization or morality, or for not advocating for legalization if recommendations were being crafted. Others might say we have taken a position "for," just by virtue of speaking to "how." What we have tried to do is benefit from the diversity of opinion in proceeding cautiously in an area of great controversy. But we wanted to proceed, to advance the debate.

In doing so, we are indebted to the authors of the papers in this volume and to the members of the Consensus Panel for their hard work, dedication, good nature, and contributions to thoughtful debate. We would also like to thank the Walter and Elise Haas Fund for support of the development of the papers in the Finding Common Ground Project series and this book, and the Wallace Alexander Gerbode Foundation for support of the project.

Clarity in bioethics, for some, is hard to find. But, at the end of the day, we often must act. Physician-assisted suicide is one of the issues in medicine and bioethics that will define who we are and want to be as individuals and as a society. We hope that this book will help to achieve at least a small measure of clarity on these issues.

Lois Snyder, J.D., Adjunct Assistant Professor of Bioethics
Arthur L. Caplan, Ph.D., Director
University of Pennsylvania Center for Bioethics

REFERENCES

1. *Washington v. Glucksberg*, 117 S.Ct. 2258 (1997); and *Vacco v. Quill*, 117 S.Ct. 2293 (1997).
2. *Oregon Death with Dignity Act*, Oregon Revised Statutes 127.800–127.897.
3. A. E. Chin et al. "Legalized Physician-Assisted Suicide in Oregon—The First Year's Experience," *New England Journal of Medicine* 340 (1999): 577–583; and A. D. Sullivan, K. Hedberg, and D. W. Fleming, "Legalized Physician-Assisted Suicide in Oregon—The Second Year," *New England Journal of Medicine* 342 (2000): 598–604.
4. Ibid.
5. L. Snyder and A. L. Caplan, eds., "Assisted Suicide: Finding Common Ground," *Annals of Internal Medicine* 132 (2000): 468–499; and D. Orentlicher and L. Snyder, "Can Assisted Suicide Be Regulated?" *Journal of Clinical Ethics* 11, no. 4 (2001): 358–366. Some of the material in this book is adapted from these articles.

One

KATRINA HEDBERG, M.D., M.P.H., AND SUSAN W. TOLLE, M.D.

Physician-Assisted Suicide and Changes in Care of the Dying: The Oregon Perspective

Introduction

The Oregon Death with Dignity Act legalizes physician-assisted suicide for terminally ill Oregon residents.[1] The act, a citizens' initiative, was first passed by Oregon voters in November 1994 by a margin of 51 percent in favor and 49 percent opposed. Immediate implementation was delayed by a legal injunction. After multiple legal proceedings, including a petition that was denied by the United States Supreme Court, the Ninth Circuit Court of Appeals lifted the injunction on 27 October 1997. On that date physician-assisted suicide became a legal, medical option for terminally ill patients in Oregon. In November 1997, Measure 51 (authorized by Oregon House Bill 2954) was placed on the general election ballot and asked Oregon voters to repeal the Death with Dignity Act. Voters chose to retain the act by a margin of 60 percent to 40 percent.

The Oregon Health Division (OHD) of the Department of Human Services and Oregon Health Sciences University's Center for Ethics in Health Care are neutral in the debate over physician-assisted suicide. In this chapter we present data on studies that have been conducted relevant to the broader changes in care of the dying in Oregon. In addition to data on the climate in Oregon surrounding physician-assisted suicide, we review the OHD data from the first two years' experience. We do not attempt to respond to criticisms of physician-assisted suicide or the act itself, or whether or not it can be ethically implemented or effectively regulated.

Background: Studies of the Climate in Oregon Prior to Implementation of Physician-Assisted Suicide

Three years elapsed between the first vote in 1994 and implementation of the Oregon Death with Dignity Act in the fall of 1997. During that period three studies were conducted by Oregon investigators examining the views of both patients and physicians toward physician-assisted suicide. These studies shed light on the attitudes and practices regarding physician-assisted suicide and end-of-life care in Oregon during the years prior to implementation.

The first study, on physicians' attitudes and practices regarding physician-assisted suicide, was conducted by Melinda Lee and colleagues in 1995 and was published in early 1996.[2] This study surveyed nearly 4,000 Oregon physicians in specialties eligible to serve as the attending physician under the act and had a 70 percent response rate. Sixty percent of responding physicians thought physician-assisted suicide should be legal in some cases. Nearly half (46 percent) indicated that they might be willing to prescribe a lethal dose of medication if the legal injunctions were lifted. More than 500 respondents (21 percent) had received a request from a patient for physician-assisted suicide during the prior year. One hundred eighty-seven doctors had written a prescription knowing the patient intended to use it to take his or her own life. This base rate of 4–7 percent is similar to that found by other investigators.

The second study was conducted by Linda Ganzini and colleagues with data collected between September 1995 and April 1997.[3] Study investigators interviewed patients with amyotrophic-lateral sclerosis (ALS) and their family caregivers exploring their attitudes toward physician-assisted suicide. All interviews were completed prior to implementation of the Death with Dignity Act. One hundred ALS patients were interviewed; fifty-six indicated that they would consider physician-assisted suicide. While many indicated that they would request lethal medication (if legal injunctions were lifted), only one patient indicated that the medication would be taken immediately. Others indicated that they would keep it for future use. Those willing to consider physician-assisted suicide were more likely to have a higher level of education and less likely to be religious.

A third study examining end-of-life care in Oregon entailed collecting data in late 1996 and throughout 1997.[4] A total of 475 family members of deceased Oregonians were interviewed from a random sample of Oregon death certificates. This study found continued progress in a broader understanding of several aspects of care of the dying in Oregon. For example, 67 percent of those who died were reported to have had a living will at the time of death. Decisions not to start treatment (79 percent) were far more common than decisions to stop treatment (21 percent). Only 2.4 percent of families reported that "too little" treatment was given.

Requirements of the Death with Dignity Act

The Oregon Death with Dignity Act was implemented in November 1997. The act allows for terminally ill Oregon residents to receive from their physician a prescription for self-administered lethal medications. The law legalizes physician-assisted suicide but specifically prohibits euthanasia (whereby a physician would directly administer a medication to end a person's life). To obtain a prescription for lethal medications in Oregon, a requesting patient must be an adult, at least eighteen years old, and a resident of Oregon. The act requires that the patient be "capable" (defined as being able to make and communicate health care decisions). The patient must have a terminal illness and have fewer than six months to live, and the request for a lethal prescription must be voluntary.

A patient who meets these requirements must make one written and two verbal requests to his or her physician. The verbal requests must be separated by at least fifteen days. The prescribing physician and a consulting physician are required to confirm the terminal diagnosis and prognosis, determine that the patient is capable and acting voluntarily, and refer the patient for counseling if either believes that the patient's judgment is impaired by a psychiatric or psychological disorder. The prescribing physician must also inform the patient of feasible alternatives such as comfort care, hospice care, and pain control options. Patients and physicians who adhere to the requirements of the act are protected from criminal prosecution.

The Task Force to Improve the Care of Terminally Ill Oregonians

The initial passage of the Death with Dignity Act catalyzed the Oregon Health Sciences University's Center for Ethics in Health Care to convene the Task Force to Improve the Care of Terminally Ill Oregonians. The task force is a consortium of health professionals, organizations, agencies, and institutions which seek to promote excellent care of the dying and to address the ethical and clinical issues posed by the enactment of the Death with Dignity Act. While individual task force members and the organizations they represent have differing views and values regarding physician-assisted suicide and the Death with Dignity Act, the task force has endeavored to maintain a neutral position on these issues. The task force convened in 1995 and has published two guide-books. The first, *The Final Months of Life: A Guide to Oregon Resources*, is a listing of approximately 800 resources in end-of-life care by county. The second, a ninety-one-page guidebook, is titled *The Oregon Death with Dignity Act: A Guidebook for Health Care Providers*.[5]

The task force spent three years in the process of writing, revising, and consensus building prior to publication and release of the guide-book for health care providers in March 1998. This fifteen-chapter guidebook begins by exploring the meaning behind a patient's request and encourages exploring concerns such as unmet pain needs or de-pression. A recent survey of physicians in Oregon regarding their ex-periences with physician-assisted suicide found that if these needs are adequately addressed, some patients no longer choose to proceed with physician-assisted suicide.[6] Another chapter explores the issue of con-scientious practice. This chapter encourages respect for the rights of all health care providers, including pharmacists, who do not wish to be involved in physician-assisted suicide. In addition to protecting the rights of those who find physician-assisted suicide morally objection-able, the task force encourages respect for the privacy of patients and providers who choose to participate.

Additional chapters outline hospice services and benefits in detail, explore patients' rights and responsibilities, and address the needs and concerns of families. For those physicians who wish to proceed with physician-assisted suicide, an extensive chapter on the role and obligations of the attending and consulting physician is provided, along with detailed information on reporting requirements to the OHD (www.ohd.hr.state.or.us/chs/pas/pas.htm). The guidebook provides general pharmacy information but does not provide a specific proto-col. The task force has recently revised the guidebook to address mi-nor modifications in Oregon statutes and to update with relevant in-formation acquired since the act's implementation. The full text of the guidebook is available on the center's Web site, www.ohsu.edu/ethics/guide.htm.

The Oregon Health Division's Role

The law requires the OHD to collect information on the patients and physicians who participate in the Death with Dignity Act, monitor com-pliance with the law, and publish an annual statistical report. To fulfill this mandate, the OHD enacted reporting rules[7] and created reporting forms. To be in compliance with the law (and to be protected from criminal prosecution), physicians are required to report all prescrip-tions for lethal medications by either completing a set of forms (avail-able from the OHD Web site) or providing copies of relevant portions of the patient's chart. For the annual reports, the OHD compiled data from these physician prescription reports and from patients' death certificates.

Because of the highly charged debate surrounding this issue, the OHD believed it was important to provide more than just a descriptive characterization of the Death with Dignity Act participants. To this end, the OHD also collected information by conducting in-depth interviews with each prescribing physician after receipt of each patient's death certificate, to learn more about patients who participated in the Death with Dignity Act. Each physician was first asked if his or her patient took the lethal medications and was then asked a series of questions about the patient's underlying illness, insurance status, and end-of-life care and concerns. During the second year the OHD continued interviewing physicians and also interviewed family members of participating patients who died between 15 September and 15 October 1999 to better understand patients' motivations for requesting physician-assisted suicide.

The OHD also compared terminally ill Oregonians who chose physician-assisted suicide and took their lethal medications with Oregonians who died from similar terminal illnesses but did not participate in the Death with Dignity Act. This comparison had two goals. The first was to understand better where physician-assisted suicide participants fit within the spectrum of all terminally ill patients in Oregon. The second was to try to address some of the questions and concerns surrounding this issue. Who would choose physician-assisted suicide and why? Would physician-assisted suicide be disproportionately chosen by patients who were poor, less educated, uninsured, fearful of financial ruin, or lacking in access to end-of-life care or proper pain control?

In constructing the reporting system and comparison study, the OHD struggled with what specific questions and issues to address. The choice of physician-assisted suicide could be influenced by moral, ethical, medical, or financial factors. The OHD chose to focus on issues that government and public health might influence such as access to hospice care, palliative pain control, lack of insurance, or financial fears. The OHD did not specifically examine the influence of moral, ethical, or religious views of the choice of physician-assisted suicide.

The First Two Years' Experience

The findings of the first two years have been published as reports, available on the OHD Web site (www.ohd.hr.state.or.us/chs/pas/ar-index. htm), and as articles in the *New England Journal of Medicine* (findings from the third year have also become available at those sources since the writing of this chapter, and are consistent with the data from the first two years).[8] The key findings from the first two years are as follows.

During 1998 the OHD received information on twenty-four persons who received prescriptions for lethal medications under the Death with Dignity Act in 1998 (no prescriptions were written under the act in 1997). Of these twenty-four prescription recipients, sixteen chose physician-assisted suicide and died after taking their lethal medications, six died from their underlying illnesses, and two were alive as of 1 January 1999). The sixteen persons who chose physician-assisted suicide accounted for 6 of every 10,000 deaths in Oregon in 1998. During 1999 thirty-three prescriptions were written for lethal doses of medication; twenty-six of these individuals took the medications, five died from their underlying illnesses, and two were alive as of 1 January 2000). One of the 1998 prescription recipients took the medications in 1999, so a total of twenty-seven patients died during 1999 as a result of physician-assisted suicide. This corresponds to 9 of every 10,000 deaths in Oregon in 1999.

The demographic and medical characteristics of patients who participated in both years were similar. The median age of the forty-three patients was seventy years; 98 percent were white; 56 percent were male; and 37 percent were college graduates. Whereas only 12 percent of the 1998 patients were married, 44 percent of the 1999 patients were married. Most patients during both years had cancer (31 or 72 percent), four had ALS, and five had chronic obstructive pulmonary disease (three had other terminal illnesses). The majority of patients were enrolled in hospice (76 percent); all but one had health insurance. Patients who chose physician-assisted suicide were comparable to all Oregonians who died of similar underlying illnesses with respect to age, race, sex, and Portland residence. However, college graduates were six times more likely to participate in physician-assisted suicide than were persons who had less than a college education.

Physicians and family members reported a variety of reasons that patients had requested physician-assisted suicide. Primary concerns expressed to physicians included loss of autonomy (79 percent); decreasing ability to participate in activities that make life enjoyable (77 percent); and loss of control of bodily functions (58 percent). No patient expressed concern about the financial consequences of treating or prolonging their illness. Family members reported similar patient concerns. In addition, physicians reported that 32 percent of patients were concerned specifically about pain. However, because some family members had difficulty separating pain from other aspects of physical suffering (for example, dyspnea, dysphagia, and medication side effects), the OHD did not distinguish pain from physical suffering in assessing family responses. Family members reported that 53 percent of patients had concerns about the more broadly defined physical suffering. Although not part of the structured interview, family members of three-fourths of the patients volunteered that the patient was determined to control the manner and circumstances surrounding his or her death.

Patients who chose physician-assisted suicide were *not* disproportionately poor (as measured by Medicaid status), less educated, lacking in insurance coverage, lacking in access to hospice care, fearful of intractable end-of-life pain, or concerned about the financial impact of their illnesses. Rather, the choice of physician-assisted suicide was most strongly associated with concerns about loss of autonomy and loss of control of bodily functions, as well as a determination to control the timing and manner of death.

Study Limitations

Several limitations should be kept in mind when one considers these findings. First, the small number of patients who chose physician-assisted suicide in 1998 and 1999 limits the ability to detect smaller differences in the characteristics of patients who chose it and those who did not. Second, the possibility of physician and family recall bias must be considered. Because of the unique nature and requirements of the Death with Dignity Act, prescribing physicians may have recalled their conversations with requesting patients in greater detail than did physicians for patients in the comparison group. The family members who were interviewed were identified by health care providers as those who knew about the patient's decision to use physician-assisted suicide and were involved in the patient's health care decisions. These family members may have had different recollections of the patient's concerns than other family members who weren't interviewed. Finally, although the OHD has no formal enforcement role, it is required to report any noncompliance with the law to the Oregon Board of Medical Examiners for further investigation. Because of this obligation, the OHD may not detect underreporting by physicians.

Recent Changes in Care of the Dying in Oregon

The process of voting, intense media campaigns, and an overall spotlight on care of the dying in Oregon have led to increased attention to end-of-life care in several ways. Oregon has the lowest rate of in-hospital deaths of the fifty states (31 percent).[9] Advance care planning occurs more frequently in Oregon than in most other states. For example, "Do

Not Resuscitate" orders were written in the charts of 91 percent of nursing home residents in one study.[10]

Pain management may also be improving for some dying patients in Oregon. In the 1997 family study, investigators asked family members about pain and suffering; 34 percent indicated that their loved one had experienced moderate to severe pain in the final week of life.[11] It is difficult to find comparable data that match this study. The only comparison data come from the national Study to Understand Prognoses and Preferences for Outcomes and Risks of Treatment (SUPPORT), which indicates that 50 percent of cognitively aware dying patients experienced moderate to severe pain in the final days of life.[12] In addition, the Oregon Board of Medical Examiners is putting increased pressure on physicians to appropriately prescribe medication to address the suffering of dying patients. In September 1999 the Oregon Board of Medical Examiners became the first in the country to discipline a physician for undertreating pain and suffering in six seriously ill and dying patients. This board has formally adopted a policy of equally investigating physicians for grossly over- or underprescribing controlled substances in their care of the dying. It is too early to assess the full implications of this action on prescribing practices in Oregon.

The Center for Ethics in Health Care has been conducting research for more than a decade tracking trends on an array of important indicators in end-of-life care. During this time steady progress has been made in such areas as increased use of hospice, the development of comfort care teams, an increased number of continuing education programs and new curricula in end-of-life care, rising rates of morphine use, falling rates of in-hospital deaths, and increasing use of and respect for advance directives.

All but one indicator remained stable or were noted to improve in all of the center's research to date. The one exception comes from interviews with family members following a loved one's death. Throughout 1997 interviews were conducted with 475 family members who were listed as the informant on the death certificate. Careful examination of these reports of loved ones' experiences near the time of death revealed one change over time.[13] Among the fifty-eight questions was one asking family members to quantify their loved one's pain in the final week of life (as comfortable, mild pain and distress, moderate pain and distress, or severe pain and distress). Whereas family members of those dying at home and in nursing homes continued to report rates of moderate or severe pain at approximately 34 percent throughout 1997, those whose loved ones died in the hospital reported rates of moderate and severe pain that increased from 33 percent in early and mid-1997 to 57 percent in the fall of 1997.[14] A follow-up study interviewing family members of those who had died in the fall of 1998 also reported higher rates of moderate to severe pain at 54 percent.[15] This second study confirms that this worrisome finding continues over time but does not explain cause and effect. A survey of Oregon physicians and nurses indicated three contributing factors in increased reports of pain in dying hospitalized patients: higher expectations, reduced physician prescribing, and reduced nurse administration.[16] Continued research is needed to better understand this finding and continue to follow important changes over time.

Future Considerations

The authors of this chapter represent the Center for Ethics in Health Care and the OHD and participate actively in gathering information about care of the dying and physician-assisted suicide in Oregon. In gathering these data, we intend to portray as accurately as possible what is happening in end-of-life care in Oregon without taking a stand on the moral issue of physician-assisted suicide and whether it is right or wrong for Oregon or for other states. We will continue to gather and publish information and in so doing will continue to protect the privacy of health care providers, patients, and their families.

The goal of the OHD is to be completely neutral in the debate over physician-assisted suicide. Maintaining neutrality and protecting the confidentiality of the patients and physicians who participate in the Death with Dignity Act are paramount if this reporting system and the resulting data are to remain legitimate. The OHD is charged with collecting data and has tried to present these data objectively and within the context of some of the ongoing debates. Nonetheless, questions remain regarding care of the dying in Oregon.

REFERENCES

1. *Oregon Death with Dignity Act*, Oregon Revised Statutes 127.800 et seq.
2. M. A. Lee et al., "Legalizing Assisted Suicide—Views of Physicians in Oregon," *New England Journal of Medicine* 334 (1996): 310–315.
3. L. Ganzini et al., "Attitudes of Patients with Amyotrophic Lateral Sclerosis and Their Care Givers toward Assisted Suicide," *New England Journal of Medicine* 339 (1998): 967–973.
4. S. W. Tolle et al., "Oregon's Low In-Hospital Death Rates: What Determines Where People Die and Satisfaction with Decisions on Place of Death?" *Annals of Internal Medicine* 130 (1999): 681–685.
5. K. Haley and M. Lee, eds., *The Oregon Death with Dignity Act: A Guidebook for Health Care Providers* (Portland: Oregon Health Sciences University, 1998).

6. L. Ganzini et al., "Physicians' Experiences with the Oregon Death with Dignity Act," *New England Journal of Medicine* 342 (2000): 557–563.
7. Oregon Administrative Rule 333-009-0000 through 333-009-0030.
8. A. E. Chin et al., "Legalized Physician-Assisted Suicide in Oregon—The First Year's Experience," *New England Journal of Medicine* 340 (1999): 577–583; and A. D. Sullivan, K. Hedberg, and D. W. Fleming, "Legalized Physician-Assisted Suicide in Oregon—The Second Year," *New England Journal of Medicine* 342 (2000): 598–604; and A. D. Sullivan, K. Hedberg, and D. Hopkins, "Legalized Physician-Assisted Suicide in Oregon, 1998–2000," *New England Journal of Medicine* 344 (2001): 605–606.
9. Tolle et al., "Oregon's Low In-Hospital Death Rates."
10. S. W. Tolle et al., "A Prospective Study of the Efficacy of the Physician Order Form for Life-Sustaining Treatment," *Journal of the American Geriatrics Society* 46 (1998): 1097–1102.
11. S. W. Tolle et al., "Family Reports of Barriers to Optimal Care of the Dying," *Nursing Research* 49 (2000): 310–317.
12. The SUPPORT Principal Investigators, "Controlled Trial to Improve the Care of Seriously-Ill Hospitalized Patients," *Journal of the American Medical Association* 274 (1995): 1591–1598.
13. Tolle et al., "Family Reports of Barriers."
14. Ibid.
15. S. W. Tolle et al., "Family Reports of Pain in Dying Hospitalized Patients: A Structured Telephone Survey," *Western Journal of Medicine* 172 (2000): 374–377.
16. S. E. Hickman et al., "Physicians' and Nurses' Perspectives on Increased Family Reports of Pain in Dying Hospitalized Patients," *Journal of Palliative Medicine* 3 (2000): 413–418.

Two

FRANKLIN G. MILLER, PH.D., JOSEPH J. FINS, M.D., AND LOIS SNYDER, J.D.

Assisted Suicide and Refusal of Treatment: Valid Distinction or Distinction without a Difference?

Introduction

SUICIDE AND ATTEMPTED SUICIDE are no longer illegal in this country. Society, however, does seek to prevent suicide, by allowing others to intervene to prevent acts of self-destruction under mental health laws and through criminalization of the act of aiding a suicide.

In recent years assisting the suicide of dying persons has become a prominent issue of public and professional debate. Although the United States Supreme Court, in June 1997, affirmed the constitutionality of laws prohibiting assisted suicide, the State of Oregon has recently implemented a law, passed by referendum, permitting physician-assisted suicide. Clarity in addressing the contested ethical and public policy issues concerning assisted suicide depends on understanding the nature of assisted suicide and how it is similar to or different from other end-of-life medical practices.

What is assisted suicide? This is a seemingly simple question. But it entails an array of questions and issues that elude easy answers. Most basically, assisted suicide is helping an individual to end his or her life. Physician-assisted suicide involves the participation of a physician in providing, but not directly administering, the medical means to help a patient perform a life-taking act. This act usually is accomplished by the patient's taking a lethal dosage of medication prescribed by a physician for that purpose.[1]

Physician-assisted suicide is one of a spectrum of end-of-life issues in the medical context, ranging from withholding or withdrawing life-sustaining treatment when patients refuse such treatment, to prescribing high doses of pain-relieving medication that risk hastening death, to active euthanasia in which a physician brings about death directly by administering a lethal injection at the request of a patient.[2] For ethical and policy analysis, it is important to try to clarify the relevant differences between these end-of-life practices, which tend to be obscured by vague and potentially misleading terminology, such as "passive euthanasia," "double-effect euthanasia," and "aid-in-dying." However, because of moral complexity and ideological conflict, clarity is difficult to achieve in this area, often resulting in confusion about end-of-life decisions[3] and decision making.

We explore here the question: Is physician-assisted suicide by ingesting prescribed lethal medication fundamentally distinct from the patient's legal and moral right to refuse life-sustaining treatment? Or is this an arbitrary distinction that is unjustly used to permit some, but not all, persons to exercise their right to determine the timing and circumstances of their death? Are there practical reasons for maintaining this distinction, despite theoretical disputes about its cogency?

In an atmosphere of intense debate over assisted suicide, culminating in the U.S. Supreme Court's recent decision that laws prohibiting assisted suicide do not violate the Constitution, the answers to these broader questions have been unclear to some and contested by others. The Second Circuit Court of Appeals based its decision to overturn New York State's law prohibiting assisted suicide as applied to competent, terminally ill patients on a rejection of the distinction between withdrawing life-sustaining treatment and assisted suicide: "Withdrawal of life support requires physicians or those acting at their direction physically to remove equipment and, often, to administer palliative drugs which may themselves contribute to death. The ending of life by these means is nothing more nor less than assisted suicide."[4] The U.S. Supreme Court, in Chief Justice William Rehnquist's majority opinion, categorically rejected this conflation of withdrawal of life-sustaining treatment and assisted suicide: "By permitting everyone to refuse unwanted medical treatment while prohibiting anyone from assisting a suicide, New York law follows a longstanding and rational distinction."[5]

Although as a matter of law the distinction between withdrawing life-sustaining treatment and assisted suicide has been reaffirmed, its conceptual and ethical validity merits exploration. In this chapter we examine critically the major reasons for and against maintaining a distinction between refusal of life-sustaining treatment and physician-assisted suicide by ingesting lethal medication. Three cases help to focus the discussion.

Illustrative Cases

Timothy Quill's narrative of the death of his patient called "Diane" has been recognized as a paradigm case of physician-assisted suicide.[6] Shortly after being diagnosed with leukemia and refusing aggressive treatment, Diane requested and received from her physician a prescription of barbiturates to be used to end her life if she determined that her suffering had become unbearable. She was enrolled in hospice. After several months, facing increasingly distressing pain, fatigue, and deterioration, she ended her life by ingesting the barbiturates.

BB, a thirty-seven-year-old woman, experienced a devastating stroke causing locked-in syndrome.[7] She became quadriplegic and was unable to speak but retained higher mental functions and perception of pain. In a rehabilitation facility BB was weaned from a ventilator and learned to communicate via a specially designed computer system. The patient, finding her quality of life intolerable, repeatedly communicated a wish to die by discontinuing artificial nutrition and hydration. Psychiatric consultation determined that she had decision-making capacity. The medical staff reluctantly agreed to withdraw life-sustaining treatment and provide comfort care for BB. Local hospices refused to accept the patient for terminal care—they said that it would constitute assisted suicide.

David Eddy, a physician and professor of health policy and management, wrote a moving narrative of his mother's death by forgoing food and water.[8] Mrs. Eddy, at age eighty-four, became bedridden, incontinent, subject to deteriorating eyesight, and confined to a nursing home after a cascade of acute medical problems. She was not dying but had irreversibly lost her capacity for independent living. Mrs. Eddy felt that she had lived a full life. She decided to seek death because of what she considered to be a drastic deterioration in her quality of life. She considered but rejected clandestine assisted suicide by ingesting lethal medication. After surviving a bout of pneumonia, despite refusing antibiotics, she chose to stop eating and drinking. Her physician agreed to help keep her comfortable while she awaited death, which arrived several days later.

Are the deaths of BB and Mrs. Eddy sufficiently similar in their circumstances to that of Diane, such that we should reject as morally arbitrary the line between refusing treatment and assisted suicide? Or are there morally significant differences between these and other comparable cases that support maintaining the line?

Reasons for Drawing the Line

Legal and ethical commentators, including Chief Justice William Rehnquist, often cite a difference of causation to account for the distinction between withdrawing life-sustaining treatment and assisted suicide.[9] Stopping life support is said to allow the patient to die by "letting nature take its course." The cause of death is not the withdrawal of treatment but the underlying disease. By contrast, in assisted suicide the cause of death is the ingestion of lethal medication prescribed by a physician.

But withdrawal of life-sustaining treatment occurs in different contexts. For patients who are imminently dying and whose lives are being prolonged temporarily by life support, it is reasonable to hold that it is the disease and not the withdrawal that is causally responsible for the patient's death. In these cases, continued treatment serves more to prolong dying than to preserve life, since death will eventuate shortly regardless of treatment. Is the situation different in cases where long-term survival is contingent on life-sustaining treatment? Though not terminally ill, BB, patients with end-stage renal disease on chronic dialysis, and ventilator-dependent patients with quadriplegia may live for years with continued life-sustaining treatment. When such patients decide to stop this treatment, the causal explanation for their deaths arguably includes both the underlying disease or injury and the withdrawal; without the withdrawal, the patients would likely have lived for extended periods of time. The right to refuse treatment, however, is not dependent on a diagnosis of terminal illness—a condition difficult to prognosticate accurately.[10]

Some have argued in favor of recognizing that withdrawals of life-support cause death by invoking the following thought experiment.[11] Suppose that a ventilator-dependent patient not seeking death was maliciously withdrawn from the ventilator by a person who plots the patient's death. The perpetrator would be charged with killing the patient and would not be able to argue successfully that "it was the underlying disease that caused the patient's death, not my pulling the plug." The malicious withdrawal causes death by the same treatment-terminating act that leads to death in the case of a competent patient who refuses continued life-sustaining treatment. It is important, however, to avoid a mistaken inference from this account of causation. Causation in fact is not the same as causation in the law. Because the conduct of clinicians in withdrawing life-sustaining treatment may in fact contribute causally to the death of patients who refuse such treatment, it does not follow that they are culpable legally or morally for wrongful killing.

Similar considerations hold for the cause of death following the forgoing of food and water. Patients who are imminently dying from a progressive disease such as cancer become cachectic and often lose their appetite for food and the urge to drink as part of the natural course of the disease.[12] If, on the verge of death, these patients stop eating and drinking, it is reasonable to attribute their death to their underlying disease. Mrs. Eddy, however, was not terminally ill. She died from dehydration subsequent to her resolute decision to stop eating and drinking.

A second commonly cited rationale for drawing the line points to a difference in physicians' intentions.[13] In the case of assisted suicide, it is claimed that the physician intends to assist in causing death by supplying the means of terminating life. In contrast, physicians who withdraw life-sustaining treatment in response to patients' refusals are considered to have fundamentally different intentions: e.g., to respect patients' rights, to relieve suffering, to stop treatment regarded as futile. Without a specific intent to help the patient terminate his or her life, clinicians do not engage in assisted suicide.

Does the complexity of end-of-life decisions support this simplistic contrast?[14] In many cases of treatment withdrawal, the intent of involved clinicians is not to bring about death. Moreover, death does not necessarily result when life-sustaining treatment is stopped. In some cases, however, the physician intends to help the patient find a way out of an irreversibly intolerable condition. Is this intent comparable to assisting in suicide by prescribing lethal medication? Both patient and physician may see treatment withdrawal resulting in death as making the best of a bad situation. On the other hand, in prescribing lethal medication at the request of a dying patient, the physician may or may not intend that the patient use it to end life. In some cases, the intent may be to provide the patient with the security of a self-administered means of ending life in response to intolerable suffering, which may help in enabling the patient to endure rather than to hasten death. Yet regardless of intent, a physician who complies with a patient's request for prescribing a lethal dose of medication is responsible for assisting in suicide if the patient takes the medication to end his or her life. Given this complexity, potential ambiguity, and the difficulty of specifying clinicians' intentions, appeal to intention offers no clear basis for a clear moral distinction between withdrawal or withholding of life-sustaining treatment and physician-assisted suicide.

Reasons for Rejecting the Line

The major criticism of a sharp distinction between withdrawing life-sustaining treatment or forgoing food and water and assisted suicide is that it is arbitrary.[15] This was a key premise in the Second Circuit Court opinion declaring that New York State's law prohibiting assisted suicide violates the equal protection clause of the Constitution's Fourteenth Amendment.[16] According to this line of argument, if cases such as those of Diane, BB, and Mrs. Eddy are viewed without legal and ethical pre-conceptions, the similarities appear at least as salient as the differences. Neither BB nor Mrs. Eddy was terminally ill. Since both patients could live for a considerable period of time, with continued treatment or by continuing to eat and drink, their decisions to stop life-sustaining treat-ment or taking food and water reflected an intent to bring about death, and these decisions causally contributed to the occurrence of death. Hence, both these cases may be accurately described as suicides.[17] In the case of Mrs. Eddy, this conclusion is further supported by the fact that she seriously contemplated assisted suicide by ingesting lethal medication. She rejected this option not because of any compunction about taking her own life but because she found distasteful the clan-destine means and the need for a plastic bag to assure the desired re-sult. Moreover, in these cases clinicians facilitated or helped accomplish the patient's intent to seek death (suicide) by withdrawing life-sustain-ing treatment (in the case of BB) and providing comfort care (in both cases). Finally, the moral considerations in favor of complying with BB's refusal of treatment and Mrs. Eddy's forgoing food and water—patient self-determination and relief of suffering—are just as relevant in the case of Diane's assisted suicide by ingesting lethal medication.[18]

Let us grant for the sake of the argument that the deaths of BB and Mrs. Eddy were suicides, provided that "suicide" is understood neu-trally without any implication of wrongdoing or motivation by an un-sound mind.[19] Does it follow that the clinicians involved in these cases were assisting in suicide? The intentional and active participation of clinicians in patients' plans to seek death would seem to be a prereq-uisite for classifying their conduct as assisted suicide. In the case of BB, the responsible clinicians resisted the patient's choice of ending her life, sought unsuccessfully to have her discharged from the rehabilita-tion facility, and complied reluctantly with refusal of treatment, recog-nizing with the help of ethics consultation that they had no right to impose treatment over the refusal of a patient who was capable of mak-ing decisions.

The inference from the patient's suicide to the clinician's assistance in suicide seems just as dubious in the case of Mrs. Eddy. The narrative of her death does not go into detail concerning the stance of her at-tending physician; it suggests that he was not actively involved in form-ing the plan of seeking death by stopping eating and drinking but was prepared to provide palliative support. Clinicians who continue to pro-vide comfort care for a competent patient who refuses food and water are treating symptoms of the underlying disease, as well as those resulting from refraining from eating and drinking; in doing so, they are not intentionally aiding in causing the patient's death.[20]

Nevertheless, the conceptual boundaries of assisted suicide are unclear, and the roles of clinicians in cases where patients seek death are subject to varying interpretations.[21] On the one hand, from a theoretical perspective, some (but certainly not all) cases of withdrawing life-sustaining treatment and forgoing food and water might be reasonably classified as assisted suicide.[22] On the other hand, practical considerations, discussed below, suggest the inappropriateness of labeling cases such as those of BB and Mrs. Eddy as "assisted suicide." Yet whether or not such cases are classified as assisted suicide, they lie within the scope of the patient's right to refuse treatment.

Refusals and Requests

There is another rationale for distinguishing withdrawing life-sustaining treatment and forgoing food and water from assisted suicide, apart from the conventional markers of causation and intent. It appeals to the morally relevant difference between refusals of life-sustaining treatment and requests for lethal medication.[23] Physicians are morally and legally required to comply with a voluntary, informed refusal of life-sustaining treatment by a competent patient, since there is no authorization for treatment without initial and continuing informed consent. A valid refusal is sufficient to authorize the withdrawal of treatment, regardless of clinicians' judgments concerning its medical or moral appropriateness. In other words, the right to refuse life-sustaining treatment ultimately functions as a trump, morally and legally obligating the compliance of responsible clinicians. To be sure, clinicians must determine that refusals of treatment are valid: i.e., they represent the voluntary, informed choices of patients who are capable of making decisions. They have a right, and possibly a duty, to advocate in favor of continued treatment, when judged medically appropriate. But once they are assured that the patient has made a valid refusal, clinicians are morally required to withhold or withdraw the refused treatment regardless of whether they judge the patient's choice to be good or bad. If, however, clinicians have moral or religious objections to honoring the patient's valid refusal, they can transfer the patient to another clinician who is prepared to uphold the patient's right of refusal.

Voluntary and informed requests by competent patients for lethal medication do not similarly obligate clinicians' compliance. Such a request is never by itself sufficient to authorize assisting in suicide. At most the request leaves compliance ethically optional, depending on the clinician's judgment of the merits of the request in view of the patient's circumstances and available alternatives. This difference is not due to the fact that withdrawal of treatment is legal whereas assisted suicide is not. Even if assisted suicide were legalized, as in Oregon, physicians would retain a right to refuse to comply with the request, because they are ethically opposed to assisted suicide or judge assisted suicide inappropriate in the circumstances faced by the patient.

Patient self-determination is much more fundamentally at stake in refusal of treatment and decisions to stop eating and drinking than in requests for lethal medication.[24] Failure to respect these former decisions by imposing unwanted medical treatment—continued life support or forced feeding and hydration—involves lack of consent to bodily invasion of a competent person, constituting a gross violation of personal freedom and rights.[25] In contrast, failure to honor a patient's voluntary request for lethal medication interferes with self-determination but does not amount to a comparable violation of the person. Individuals denied requested lethal medication remain free to seek death by stopping any life-sustaining treatment or refraining from eating and drinking. The differential moral force associated with decisions to refuse life-sustaining treatment and to forgo food and water, as compared with a request for lethal medication, counts as a morally significant reason for maintaining this distinction.

Implications of Holding the Line

Maintaining the line distinguishing withdrawal of life-sustaining treatment and forgoing food and water from assisted suicide by lethal medication has a number of significant implications for public policy and medical ethics. If refusal of life-sustaining treatment and assisted suicide are equivalent, then there would be no rational basis for the law to permit the former while prohibiting the latter. The U.S. Supreme Court firmly endorsed the distinction between refusal of treatment and assisted suicide, thus rejecting the logic of the Second Circuit Court that the state lacks any rational grounds for prohibiting assisted suicide for competent, terminally ill patients.

Maintaining the distinction, however, does not settle the issue of whether assisted suicide for competent, terminally ill patients by means of prescribed lethal medication should remain prohibited by law. The desirability of prohibition versus legalization is a matter of policy that the Court wisely left up to the states to decide by democratic means. Nevertheless, the distinction between refusal of life-sustaining treatment and assisted suicide has important policy implications for the debate over whether and how to legalize assisted suicide. Critical issues include the scope of a possible legal option of physician-assisted suicide and the nature of appropriate regulatory safeguards.

If there is no valid distinction between assisted suicide and forgoing life-sustaining treatment, then a legal option of assisted suicide should be just as broad in its scope as the right to refuse treatment. There would be no principled basis for confining assisted suicide to terminally ill patients, since the right to refuse life-sustaining treatment is available to all competent patients, regardless of prognosis.[26] Similarly, if assisted suicide and forgoing life-sustaining treatment are equivalent, then surrogate decision-makers should be permitted to authorize lethal medication for patients who lack decision-making capacity, since surrogate decision making is recognized for withholding and withdrawing treatment for such patients.

Proposals to legalize assisted suicide have generally included regulatory safeguards, such as mandatory waiting periods and consultation with palliative experts, designed to assure that the patient is making a voluntary, informed, and resolute decision and that lethal medication is used only as a measure of last resort.[27] These safeguards go beyond what is required by law for valid refusals of life-sustaining treatment. The rationale for more stringent safeguards in the case of a legal option of assisted suicide depends on upholding some form of the distinction: They are justifiable because assisted suicide by means of lethal medication is not equivalent to withdrawing life-sustaining treatment.

The distinction between refusal of treatment and assisted suicide has traditionally been understood in medical ethics as a matter of moral justification. Under this interpretation, refusals of life-sustaining treatment by competent patients, provided they are voluntary and informed, are morally valid; assisted suicide is not. However, a consensus in favor of this interpretation has eroded. Powerful arguments have been presented, appealing to patient self-determination and relief of suffering, in favor of justifying physician-assisted suicide and/or voluntary active euthanasia in response to the voluntary, informed requests of competent patients facing dire circumstances and lacking acceptable alternatives. If these arguments are sound, it does not follow that the distinction is irrelevant to medical ethics. The understanding of the line separating forgoing life-sustaining treatment and assisted suicide in terms of the difference between refusals and requests has the merit of leaving open the moral justifiability of acts of assisted suicide. Yet, as indicated above, significant moral differences remain, regardless of whether some acts of physician-assisted suicide are regarded as morally justifiable.

Practical Considerations

A number of practical considerations bolster maintaining the line between refusal of treatment and assisted suicide. As long as assisted suicide remains illegal and contrary to prevailing ethical standards for medical practice, it is confusing and awkward to classify compliance with a patient's legal right to refuse treatment or to forgo food and water as assisted suicide. More importantly, erasing or modifying the traditional line between forgoing life-sustaining treatment and assisted suicide may undermine clinicians' support for the former.[28] It was not long ago that physicians were hesitant to withdraw life support. Many clinicians continue to find withdrawal of life-sustaining treatment troubling, since it is apt to appear as an active intervention that results in a patient's death. The recognition of a legal and moral right of competent patients to refuse life-sustaining treatment has been premised on the basis that this does not amount to assisted suicide or active euthanasia.[29] For many clinicians the willingness to support and continue to care for patients who decide to withdraw life-sustaining treatment or to stop eating and drinking is likely to depend on the belief that doing so is not assisted suicide.

Another potential consequence of equating withdrawal of life-sustaining therapy with assisted suicide is that a clinician who wishes to respect the refusal of treatment but wants to avoid the perception of assisting suicide may find it necessary to disguise a withdrawal in a way that compromises his or her integrity. For example, extubation may be labeled as an effort to wean the patient from mechanical ventilation, when the patient has not met the criteria for weaning. Thus, with a DNR order in place, the clinician may withdraw ventilatory support, knowing that the patient cannot breathe independently. Resuscitative efforts will be withheld when respiratory arrest occurs.

Clinicians prepared to withdraw mechanical ventilation without engaging in such an integrity-compromising approach may still be reluctant to provide adequate sedation out of fear that this crosses the line into the territory of assisted suicide or active euthanasia. However, sedation is medically indicated to counteract "air hunger" in extubated patients who have refused continued mechanical ventilation[30] and should not be confused or conflated with administering medication for the purpose of ending the patient's life.

Conclusion

We have reviewed critically reasons for and against maintaining an ethical distinction between a competent patient's decision to forgo life-sustaining treatment or to stop eating and drinking, on the one hand, and physician-assisted suicide by ingesting a prescribed dose of lethal medication, on the other. The theoretical question about whether these end-of-life decisions are morally equivalent is likely to remain contested. Competent patients, however, have a recognized legal and moral right to refuse all life-sustaining treatment—a right that extends as well to forgoing food and water for patients capable of eating and drinking. The traditional prohibition in medical ethics of physicians prescribing or administering a lethal drug is likely to continue to influence a significant proportion of physicians, regardless of whether physician-assisted suicide is legalized. Equating cases of withdrawing life-sustaining treatment or providing palliative care to a patient who stops eating and drinking with ingesting physician-prescribed lethal medication potentially imperils physicians' support for patients' rights. Erasing the line between forgoing life-sustaining treatment and assisted suicide could set back the moral progress of the past twenty years in expanding the rights of patients to control life-and-death decisions and could undermine the care of dying patients.[31]

REFERENCES

1. M. J. Field and C. K. Cassel, eds., *Approaching Death: Improving Care at the End of Life* (Washington: National Academy Press, 1997).
2. L. Snyder and A. L. Caplan, "Die Hard: End-of-Life Care in America," *Pennsylvania Medicine* 99 (1996): 10–11; and J. J. Fins and M. D. Bacchetta, "Framing the Physician-Assisted Suicide and Voluntary Active Euthanasia Debate: The Role of Deontology, Consequentialism, and Clinical Pragmatism," *Journal of the American Geriatrics Society* 43 (1995): 563–568.
3. P. A. Ubel and D. Asch, "Semantic and Moral Debates about Hastening Death: A Survey of Bioethicists," *Journal of Clinical Ethics* 8 (1997): 242–249.
4. *Quill v. Vacco*, 80 F.3d 716,729 (1996).
5. *Vacco v. Quill*, 117 S.Ct. 2293 (1997).
6. T. E. Quill, "Death and Dignity: A Case of Individualized Decision Making," *New England Journal of Medicine* 324 (1991): 691–694.
7. T. Powell and B. Lowenstein, "Refusing Life-Sustaining Treatment after Catastrophic Injury: Ethical Implications," *Journal of Law, Medicine, and Ethics* 24 (1996): 54–61.
8. D. M. Eddy, "A Conversation with My Mother," *Journal of the American Medical Association* 272 (1994): 179–181.
9. *Vacco v. Quill*; D. Callahan, *The Troubled Dream of Life: In Search of a Peaceful Death* (New York: Simon and Schuster, 1993), 76–82; and E. D. Pellegrino, "Doctors Must Not Kill," *Journal of Clinical Ethics* 3 (1992): 95–102.
10. W. A. Knaus et al., "The SUPPORT Prognostic Model: Objective Estimates of Survival for Seriously Ill Hospitalized Adults," *Annals of Internal Medicine* 121 (1995): 191–203; and N. A. Christakis and J. J. Escarce, "Survival of Medicare Patients after Enrollment in Hospice Programs," *New England Journal of Medicine* 335 (1996): 172–178.
11. D. W. Brock, "Voluntary Active Euthanasia," in *Life and Death* (New York: Cambridge University Press, 1993), 208–213.
12. R. M. McCann, W. J. Hall, and A. Groth-Juncker, "Comfort Care for Terminally Ill Patients: The Appropriate Use of Nutrition and Hydration," *Journal of the American Medical Association* 272 (1994): 1263–1266.
13. *Vacco v. Quill*; and Christakis and Escarce, "Survival of Medicare Patients."

14. T. E. Quill, "The Ambiguity of Clinical Intentions," *New England Journal of Medicine* 329 (1993): 1039–1040.
15. J. Rachels, "Active and Passive Euthanasia," *New England Journal of Medicine* 292 (1975): 78–80.
16. *Quill v. Vacco.*
17. D. W. Brock, "Death and Dying," in *Life and Death*, 165–166.
18. Brock, "Voluntary Active Euthanasia."
19. T. L. Beauchamp, "The Problem of Defining Suicide," in *Ethical Issues in Death and Dying*, 2d ed., ed. T. L. Beauchamp and R. M. Veatch (Upper Saddle River, N.J.: Prentice Hall, 1996), 112–117.
20. F. G. Miller and D. E. Meier, "Voluntary Death: A Comparison of Terminal Dehydration and Physician-Assisted Suicide," *Annals of Internal Medicine* 128 (1998): 559–562.
21. H. Brody, "Causing, Intending, and Assisting Death," *Journal of Clinical Ethics* 4 (1993): 112–117.
22. T. L. Beauchamp and J. F. Childress, *Principles of Biomedical Ethics*, 4th ed. (New York: Oxford University Press, 1994), 238–239; and G. E. Pence, *Classic Cases in Medical Ethics*, 2d ed. (New York: McGraw Hill, 1995), 51.
23. J. L. Bernat, B. Gert, and R. P. Mogielnicki, "Patient Refusal of Hydration and Nutrition: An Alternative to Physician Assisted Suicide or Voluntary Active Euthanasia," *Archives of Internal Medicine* 153 (1993): 2723–2728.
24. F. G. Miller, "Legalizing Physician-Assisted Suicide by Judicial Decision: A Critical Appraisal," *BioLaw* (July–August 1996): S136–S145.
25. New York State Task Force on Life and the Law, *When Death Is Sought: Assisted Suicide and Euthanasia in the Medical Context* (Albany: New York State Task Force, 1994), 146–147.
26. A. Meisel, "The Legal Consensus about Forgoing Life-Sustaining Treatment: Its Status and Its Prospects," *Kennedy Institute of Ethics Journal* 2 (1992): 309–345.
27. F. G. Miller et al., "Regulating Physician-Assisted Death," *New England Journal of Medicine* 331 (1994): 119–123; and C. H. Baron et al., "A Model State Act to Authorize and Regulate Physician-Assisted Suicide," *Harvard Journal on Legislation* 33 (1996): 1–34.
28. S. M. Wolf, "Holding the Line on Euthanasia," *Hastings Center Report* 19, no. 1 (1989): S13–S15.
29. Meisel, "The Legal Consensus about Forgoing Life-Sustaining Treatment."
30. M. J. Edwards and S. W. Tolle, "Disconnecting a Ventilator at the Request of a Patient Who Knows That He Will Then Die: The Doctor's Anguish," *Annals of Internal Medicine* 117 (1992): 254–256.
31. A. Alpers and B. Lo, "Does It Make Clinical Sense to Equate Terminally Ill Patients who Require Life-Sustaining Interventions with Those Who Do Not?" *Journal of the American Medical Association* 277 (1997): 1705–1706.

Three

ARTHUR L. CAPLAN, PH.D.,

LOIS SNYDER, J.D., AND

KATHY FABER-LANGENDOEN, M.D.

The Role of Guidelines in the Practice of Physician-Assisted Suicide

Introduction

Proponents and opponents of physician-assisted suicide can agree on at least one thing: the importance of regulatory guidelines if the practice is to be legal. However, there is much disagreement about the moral import of even trying to formulate guidelines; about what effect guidelines can have on physician practice, health care providers, patients, or families; and whether any set of guidelines can really protect against harm or abuse. Questions once of theoretical interest have taken on new urgency as Oregon has moved from legalization to actual implementation of physician-assisted suicide.

The debate about guidelines swirls around a number of interrelated questions. What has been the experience of efforts to implement physician-assisted suicide using consensus guidelines? What goals are guidelines intended to serve? Who should formulate them? Can guidelines be practical? Are there obstacles to creating or implementing guidelines? And, is dying a process amenable to direction under guidelines by physicians, departments of health, blue-ribbon panels, or other regulatory bodies?

What Is Known about the Value of Guidelines for Physician-Assisted Suicide?

The Netherlands, where euthanasia and physician-assisted suicide have been decriminalized, is the only place where guidelines have existed for any significant period of time. The national medical association along with groups such as pharmacologists[1] undertook their development. Many in the American debate invoke data from the Netherlands to support their positions.[2] But there are limits to what can be learned from the Dutch experience.

The Dutch value guidelines, but while the practice was technically illegal, the force of guidelines and their precision was not what would have been expected were the practice legal. Dutch physicians noted that many physicians did not follow guidelines or do the required reporting,[3] and formal studies noted high rates of noncompliance as well.[4] The Dutch, however, have recently legalized euthanasia and physician-assisted suicide.

The facts about how well Dutch guidelines regulated the practice of physician-assisted suicide are in dispute.[5] Reports of involuntary euthanasia (causing the death of the patient without an unambiguous request to die from the patient), prompted a reexamination of prevailing guidelines. More restrictive rules with tougher reporting and witness requirements have been adopted.[6] Studies comparing practices in 1995 with those in 1990 have found that involuntary euthanasia continues to occur at a minimally lower rate. However, a large number of deaths with assistance go unreported to the authorities.[7] Thus, it is hard to draw clear lessons from the Netherlands about the effectiveness of guidelines. Differences in the health systems and social structure of the Netherlands and the United States further complicate comparisons.

What Are Guidelines For?

The first published proposals for U.S. guidelines to govern the implementation of legally sanctioned physician-assisted suicide appeared in the early 1990s. The movement to create guidelines has been a key component in efforts toward legalization and has focused on how to implement a decision to proceed with physician-assisted suicide (as opposed to how to make a decision that physician-assisted suicide is the "right" course for an individual). Some of the efforts have created model statutes or legislation. But most discussion of guidelines has focused on providing practical guidance about implementing physician-assisted suicide in an authoritative document.

Legalization is not a prerequisite for the creation of guidelines. Many who initially called for guidelines noted that the practice of physician-assisted suicide was already occurring in the United States. They argued that it would be better to have some sort of guidance for doctors rather than leaving each doctor and patient to their own devices, unmonitored. In fact, those favoring legalization felt that the cause of legalization would be advanced by promoting practical guidelines. This created a situation in which guidelines were often viewed by critics as nothing more then a stalking horse for efforts to legalize physician-assisted suicide.

Jack Kevorkian's actions and advocacy brought new urgency to guideline-writing efforts. Lonnie Shavelson[8] documented a number of cases in which he felt that persons had assisted others to die for reasons that were morally dubious. The popularity of books such as *Final Exit* and *Last Wish* made it clear there was public interest in assisted suicide and a hunger for information about how to best proceed once the decision had been made to die.[9] Yale physician Sherwin Nuland's book *How We Die* reinforced the view that all too often the prevailing standard of clinical care for the dying was not what patients and their families wanted.[10]

The inadequate state of end-of-life care was further evident in the findings of the Study to Understand Prognoses and Preferences for Outcomes and Risks of Treatment (SUPPORT).[11] It was obvious that something had to be done to standardize and improve the overall care of the dying. If nothing was done, assisted suicide might become commonplace without input from those most experienced in caring for the terminally ill.

Those calling for regulation of physician-assisted suicide often made analogies to the impact law and regulation had had on the practice of forgoing, withdrawing, and withholding life support. The willingness of society to accept the cessation of ventilators, renal dialysis, antibiotics, and other life-sustaining interventions on the basis of policies, guidelines, and review by ethics committees made many believe that what had worked effectively for forgoing life-sustaining treatment could work for physician-assisted suicide.[12]

Finally, in several opinion surveys done in the early 1990s, it became clear that many patients and doctors would consider physician-assisted suicide for reasons that experts in end-of-life care found troubling or simply erroneous.[13] Those polled said they would consider physician-assisted suicide if they were in terrible pain or had to be dependent on machines. This made some proponents think that regulation was essential, to ensure that those disabled or in pain would not seize upon physician-assisted suicide prematurely.

Who Should Write Guidelines?

Despite all of the efforts at guideline development, there has been relatively little discussion of who should create them. In Oregon, guideline development fell to the Department of Health, although guidance was also offered by the medical society[14] and a blue-ribbon panel.[15] Other groups who have issued guidelines over the years have tended to consist of professors and academics, with a few clinicians favoring legalization. They moved to formulate guidelines more from political necessity than as a function of special expertise or clinical involvement with those making requests or the terminally ill.[16] One notable exception was the Bay Area Network of Ethics Committees, which in 1997 issued guidelines to help clinicians respond to requests for assistance in dying.[17] In part, these guidelines were in response to numerous requests for physician-assisted suicide from San Francisco residents dying of acquired immune deficiency syndrome (AIDS).

Obviously, those favoring legalization are most likely to write guidelines. In the few instances in which medical groups tried to write guidelines without prior agreement about the desirability of physician-assisted suicide (Michigan Medical Society, New York Academy of Medicine), the effort collapsed.[18] Critics sometimes take on the specifics of proposed guidelines but, more often, reject guidelines on general grounds (i.e., no guidelines could ever be sufficient to prevent the inclusion of inappropriate cases)[19] or as an opportunity to engage in further debate about the general moral merits of legalization.[20] Interestingly, when proponents write guidelines, their focus is on either physicians or public policy-makers as the intended audience; not patients, the general public, or the religious community.

While religious groups have spoken to the morality of physician-assisted suicide, none has issued any specific guidelines on its implementation or monitoring.[21] The Task Force to Improve the Care of Terminally Ill Oregonians, formed to help provide guidance in implementing the Oregon law, was composed mostly of physicians, nurses, and attorneys.[22] No patient or consumer groups have issued specific guidelines. This is especially noteworthy given the growing interest in the spiritual and psychological dimensions of dying, as reflected in the enormous popularity of books focusing on these aspects of dying.[23] Guidelines have been seen for the most part as norms or rules aimed at the doctors, not more general principles about how Americans ought to think about, control, or implement physician-assisted suicide.

In fact, the American debate about assisted suicide seems to focus on the presumption that the persons who should be most concerned about implementing assisted suicide are physicians (see Chapter 4). Perhaps this stance is fueled in part by the opposition to assisted suicide by physicians or nurses on the part of organized medicine and nursing throughout the 1990s, on the grounds that such behavior violates norms of professional ethics. But the centrality of doctors as the audience for guidelines may also reflect a deeply held American view that dying is a matter with which health care professionals and biomedical science must contend.[24]

Content of Guidelines for Physician-Assisted Suicide

A sample of the guidelines reveals consistent core content (see Table 3.1). Looking at the first set of guidelines published in a major medical journal,[25] others in prominent publications,[26] and state requirements (Oregon), a number of common themes emerge. All require the individual's informed consent for participation (mental competency or capacity, awareness of options and alternatives, voluntariness). Guidelines usually recommend a waiting period to ensure the authenticity of a request. Most guidelines call for consent to be written and witnessed.

Guidelines with more physician input include references to conscientious objection. They also try to capture the importance of good doctor-patient relationships by including discussions of "meaningful" and/or established relationships. They seek to ensure that the attending physician's judgment is subjected to review by another physician to prevent error or even malice. More recent guidelines tend to include suggestions that independent specialists in palliative care review requests for physician-assisted suicide, that psychiatrists or psychologists be involved in assessing the competency of those making requests, and that palliative care not only be discussed as an alternative but actually be offered to a person making a request.

Recent guidelines confine their scope to the terminally ill, defined as those with six months or less to live. Some earlier efforts and a recent California group, however, focused on those individuals with incurable conditions and intolerable pain (as the Dutch guidelines did).[27]

Critical Reactions to Proposed Guidelines

The general concerns revealed in assessments of guidelines are that they will not work in American society because no guidelines are capable of "holding the line" with respect to limiting physician-assisted suicide to particular individuals or groups, and worries about the practical applicability of guidelines to the real world of clinical practice—slippery slopes and impracticalities.[28]

A task force in New York State argued that guidelines would "prove elastic in clinical practice and law."[29] Perhaps the harshest indictment of efforts to construct guidelines comes from Callahan and White,[30] who dismiss all efforts at constructing guidelines as "an elaborate regulatory facade concealing a poverty of potential for actual enforcement."

The main reason for thinking that the slope around physician-

Table 3.1   "Guidelines" for Implementing Physician-Assisted Suicide

Who Developed the Guideline	Title of Guideline	Disciplines Involved	Year	Areas Addressed
BANEC[a]	*Physician-Hastened Death: Advisory Guidelines for the San Francisco Bay Area from the Bay Area Network of Ethics Committees (BANEC)*	Medicine, public health, nursing	1997	Patient characteristics (must be terminally ill, defined as < 6 months to live, competent, not depressed, and making voluntary request); physician requirements (palliative care must be made available, consultation procedure, informed consent process, death certification); role of family
Baron et al.[b]	*A Model State Act to Authorize and Regulate PAS*	Medicine, law, philosophy, ethics, economics	1996	Patient characteristics (18+ years, terminally ill, i.e. < 6 months); physician requirements (palliation offered, counseling, consultation, documentation, presence at death, conscientious objection option); family role; and legal issues (confidentiality, monitoring/enforcement, and liability)
Coleman and Fleischman[c]	*Guidelines for PAS: Can the Challenge Be Met?*	Medicine, law	1996	"Un-guidelines"—evaluate existing guidelines and conclude that despite good intentions, guidelines will not be able to limit PAS to narrowly defined circumstances

Drickamer, Lee, and Ganzini[d]	*Practical Issues in PAS*	Medicine	1997	Areas of physician skill and knowledge required (understanding of patient motivation, mental states, difficulties in prognostication); role of family and of other providers; PAS methods available; and effects on patient-physician relationship
Miller et al.[e]	*Regulating Physician-Assisted Death*	Medicine, philosophy, ethics, law	1994	Patient characteristics (competent, terminal, voluntary); request prerequisites (palliative care offered and judged unsatisfactory); regulatory requirements and protections; and consultative and monitoring mechanisms (palliative care consultants and committees)
Quill, Cassel, and Meier[f]	*Care of the Hopelessly Ill: Proposed Clinical Criteria for PAS*	Medicine	1992	Patient characteristics (incurable condition, severe and unrelenting suffering, capacitated); physician requirements (established relationship, conscientious objection option, documentation requirements, and consultation process)

Table 3.1 *Continued*

Who Developed the Guideline	Title of Guideline	Disciplines Involved	Year	Areas Addressed
Task Force to Improve the Care of Terminally Ill Oregonians (with funding by the Greenwall Foundation)[g]	The Oregon Death with Dignity Act: A Guidebook for Health Care Providers	Medicine, law, nursing, pharmacy, public health, social work, hospice, state agencies, health systems	1998	Guidebook to implement the Oregon Death with Dignity Act; patient characteristics (voluntary request, 18+ years, resident of Oregon, and terminal, i.e. < 6 months); physician requirements (disclosure, process for rescinding requests, conscientious objection); and legal elements (immunity and reporting/monitoring by state)
Young et al. (with funding by the Walter and Elise Haas Fund and Wallace Alexander Gerbode Foundation)[h]	*Report of The Northern California Conference for Guidelines on Aid-in-Dying*	Medicine, ethics, nursing, law, religion	1997	Patient characteristics (terminal illness defined as incurable condition with intolerable, irremediable suffering as defined by patient; capacity, voluntariness, and other decision-making prerequisites); consultation and palliative care requirements; role of family; role of ethics committees, of institutions, and special concerns raised by managed care

Sources: See below.

[a]S. Hellig, R. Brody, F. S. Marcus, L. Shavelson, and P. C. Sussman, "Physician-Hastened Death: Guidelines for San Francisco Bay Area Network of Ethics Committees," *Western Journal of Medicine* 166 (1997): 37–78.

[b] C. H. H. Baron, C. Bergstresser, D. W. Brock, et al., "A Model State Act to Authorize and Regulate Physician-Assisted Suicide," *Harvard Journal on Legislation* 33 (1996): 1–34.

[c] C. H. Coleman and A. R. Fleischman, "Guidelines for Physician-Assisted Suicide: Can the Challenge Be Met?" *Journal of Law, Medicine, and Ethics* 24 (1996): 217–224.

[d] M. A. Drickamer, M. A. Lee, and L. Ganzini, "Practical Issues in Physician Assisted Suicide," *Annals of Internal Medicine* 126 (1997): 146–151.

[e] F. G. Miller, T. E. Quill, H. Brody, J. C. Fletcher, L. O. Gostin, and D. E. Meier, "Regulating Physician-Assisted Death," *New England Journal of Medicine* 331 (1994): 119–123.

[f] T. E. Quill, C. K. Cassell, and D. E. Meier, "Care of the Hopelessly Ill: Proposed Clinical Criteria for Physician-Assisted Suicide," *New England Journal of Medicine* 327 (1992): 1380–1384.

[g] Task Force to Improve the Care of Terminally Ill Oregonians, *The Oregon Death with Dignity Act: A Guidebook for Health Care Providers* (Portland: Oregon Health Sciences University, 1998).

[h] E. W. D. Young, F. S. Marcus, T. Dought, M. Mendiola, C. Carlucci-Ciesielski, A. Alpers, et al., "Report of the North California Conference for Guidelines on Aid-in-Dying: Definitions, Differences, Convergences, Conclusions," *Western Journal of Medicine* 166 (1997): 381–388.

assisted suicide might be too slippery even for the most carefully crafted guidelines is that the presumptions behind the guidelines are inherently slippery in ways that no amount of regulatory precision can fix. If physician-assisted suicide is to be limited to the terminally ill, problems arise from physicians' inability to accurately predict who truly is terminally ill. If physician-assisted suicide is to be limited only to those who are competent, problems arise when competency and capacity are difficult to define and assess. There may also be unwanted pressure to end one's life earlier if there is a danger that competency may evaporate as illness progresses. And if it is truly suffering as well as pain that leads persons to support physician-assisted suicide, then the category of what counts as unbearable suffering or emotional distress is flexible enough to permit and, indeed, require expansion beyond the terminally ill.

One way to respond to these sorts of concerns is to note that guidelines alone will never be sufficient to control the practice of physician-assisted suicide. As is true of any rule-based practice, there will always have to be room left for discretion and judgment. Bad people will not be stopped from doing unethical things because rules exist. But, good people can be trusted to make reasonable accommodations in the light of rules. Since decisions are made in medicine every day on the basis of decisions about terminal illness, competency, and what counts as unbearable pain or suffering, it will not suffice as an argument to say that since these are vague concepts with fuzzy borders they cannot be used to guide the practice of physician-assisted suicide if they are already in use and guiding the practice of terminating treatment, deciding whether or not to perform CPR or to enlist a person in an innovative experimental protocol to try a last-ditch therapy. Precision is important, but no set of rules—be they for the courtroom, athletic competitions, operating motor vehicles, or physician-assisted suicide—will be so precise as to permit the creation of clear, bright lines and absolute categories that eliminate all gray areas and the need for prudent judgment.

The real core of the slippery-slope objections to guidelines rests on the cost of making a mistake. If persons who do not fit the paradigm commit suicide, then what moral judgment should be made about this practice and those involved in it? For many Americans, erring on the side of physician-assisted suicide when competency is in doubt or a prognosis of terminal illness is uncertain might prove tolerable if pain and suffering were clear. However, if uncertainty regarding suffering, terminal illness, and competency is present, the moral assessment of rules that would permit errors to be made in these circumstances would be far more harsh. Both critics with slippery-slope concerns and proponents of physician-assisted suicide need to address more clearly their positions about mistakes.

The other major source of concern about guidelines is feasibility. Physicians sometimes have difficulty diagnosing and managing mental illness, depression, and delirium. In addition, they often have not had long-term relationships with their patients. Time and inexpertise can limit physicians' ability to engage in philosophical rumination or spiritual reflections with patients. Is it appropriate to ask doctors to ensure that family or financial pressures have not coerced patients into asking for physician-assisted suicide? Should physicians be asked to overcome their own moral reservations about suicide when cost pressures and new modes of health care delivery are building more and more walls between doctors and patients?

It may also be infeasible to offer persons alternatives to physician-assisted suicide in the context of American health care.[31] For many Americans, hospice or an adequate nursing home or high-quality home care are not available. With many lacking insurance and others living in areas where services are scarce or culturally insensitive, no set of rules can compensate for the absence of decent basic health care for the dying.

One other practical problem which may limit the feasibility of rules is the absence of an infrastructure for providing oversight to the dying in America. Relatively few doctors and nurses are skilled at palliative care, so developing committees of specialists to monitor clinical practice could prove a daunting task.

Other Concerns

The debate about guidelines to regulate the practice of physician-assisted suicide is shaped more by overall attitudes about the desirability or undesirability of legalizing physician-assisted suicide than by any particular set of guidelines and their virtues. In some ways, this has narrowed the discussion.

Most guidelines are written by people who come at the issue of dying from the point of view of either providers of health care or those involved in the law and regulation.[32] This may be necessary in some ways, but it contributes greatly to the sense that these guidelines are disconnected from the patient and family's world of illness, suffering, and dying and that the guidelines serve providers and payers more than patients. The way the guidelines are written has less to do with trust and collaboration between a health care provider and a patient and far more with the provision of legal indemnification.[33] It would be most interesting to see the sort of guidelines about physician-assisted suicide that would be written with contributions by persons whose partners, family members, or friends had recently died or who had themselves experienced serious chronic illness or disability. Medical and legal groups emphasize vastly different issues compared to the messages sent about the meaning and significance, pace and pattern, lessons and morals of dying contained in popular books, movies, plays, and television programs.[34]

Significantly, while many Americans turn to religious or spiritual frameworks to guide them through dying, these voices are rare in current guidelines. What is striking about the guidelines is how often they refer to the need for certainty about diagnosis, autonomy, and competency—surely major worries for providers—rather than to issues of dependency, relationships, timing, stigma, guilt, symbolism, cultural practices, funeral arrangements, money, and other matters of overwhelming concern to patients and their families.[35]

Medicine is often criticized for turning dying into a dehumanized process mediated by technologies operated by strangers. There is much about the extant guidelines that exhibits these same problems. To date, regulation looks like it is being fueled by the desire of providers to avoid error and escape liability and by the desire of lawyers to ensure that the law does not permit physician-assisted suicide to lapse into murder. Concerns about what a good death is[36] and related issues as to how one brings a narrative to a close and says goodbye to loved ones and others, along with issues of ceremonies, ritual, and prayer, for example, are not addressed. While the law might be too blunt an instrument for such matters, guidelines are not. On the other hand, a focus on guidelines may itself reveal a preoccupation with the wrong questions.

Pain control and the role of palliative care specialists[37] are crucial to good end-of-life care and areas in which health care has been deficient in this country, although that is beginning to change. They play a role in more recent guidelines. But good pain control and palliative care are not truly alternatives to those who seek a right to physician-assisted suicide in order to gain control over the manner and timing of death.

Those who oppose legalization have made much of the importance of better pain control and better palliation as alternatives. But those who face death may not be troubled by the prospect of pain (as was the case for the individuals who committed suicide with physician assistance in the first year of the Oregon law's implementation).[38] More often they are troubled by the prospect of loss of dignity as they define it, isolation, loneliness, fear, anxiety, the expectations that others have of them, the desire not to make others sorrow or grieve, and what will happen to loved ones after their death. Many do not wish to die with their minds fogged or unconscious. These matters and views of what a good death requires are not handled by the ample provision of pain-controlling medications, but they are crucial in articulating the sort of guidance that is needed to bring about a good death.[39]

While autonomy dominates the moral outlook of current guidelines, dying is rarely an isolated, autonomous event. If the good death is truly to be a part of physician-assisted suicide, or assisted suicide more broadly, existing guidelines will have to be supplemented with voices and concerns that range beyond the realm of informed consent, clinical competence, and legal liability.

REFERENCES

1. P. Pijnenborg, *End of Life Decisions in Dutch Medical Practice* (The Hague, Netherlands: CIP-Gegevens Koniglijke Bibliotheek, 1995); Commission on the Study of Medical Practice concerning Euthanasia, *Medical Decisions concerning the End of Life* (in Dutch) (The Hague: Staatsuitgeverij, 1991) (also known as "the Remmelink Report"); Royal Dutch Society for the Advancement of Pharmacology, *The Administration of and Preparation for Euthanasia* (The Hague: Royal Dutch Society, 1994); and B. Sneiderman, "Euthanasia in the Netherlands: A Model for Canada?" *Humane Medicine* 8 (1992): 104–115.

2. M. P. Battin, *The Least Worst Death: Essays in Bioethics on the End of Life* (New York: Oxford, 1994); C. Gomez, *Regulating Death: Euthanasia and the Case of the Netherlands* (New York: Free Press, 1991); and W. J. Smith, *Forced Exit: The Slippery Slope from Assisted Suicide to Legalized Murder* (New York: Times Books, 1997).

3. M. Simons, "Dutch Doctors to Tighten Rules on Mercy Killings," *New York Times*, 9 September 1995.

4. P. J. van der Maas et al., "Euthanasia, Physician-Assisted Suicide, and Other Medical Practices Involving the End of Life in the Netherlands, 1990–1995," *New England Journal of Medicine* 335 (1996): 1699–1705.

5. Pijnenborg, *End of Life Decisions in Dutch Medical Practice*; Battin, *The Least Worst Death*; Gomez, *Regulating Death*; Smith, *Forced Exit*; Simons, "Dutch Doctors to Tighten Rules on Mercy Killings"; and H. Hendin, *Seduced by Death: Doctors, Patients, and Assisted Suicide* (New York: W. W. Norton, 1998).

6. Simons, "Dutch Doctors to Tighten Rules on Mercy Killings"; and van der Maas et al., "Euthanasia, Physician-Assisted Suicide, and Other Medical Practices."

7. G. van der Wal et al., "Evaluation of the Notification Procedure for Physician-Assisted Death in the Netherlands," *New England Journal of Medicine* 335 (1996): 1706–1711.

8. L. Shavelson, *A Chosen Death: The Dying Confront Assisted Suicide* (New York: Simon and Schuster, 1995).

9. D. Humphry, *Final Exit: The Practicalities of Self-Deliverance and Assisted Suicide for the Dying* (New York: Dell Publishing, 1991); and B. Rollin, *Last Wish* (New York: Warner Books, 1985).

10. S. B. Nuland, *How We Die: Reflections on Life's Final Chapter* (New York: Knopf, 1994).

11. The SUPPORT Principal Investigators, "A Controlled Trial to Improve Care for Seriously Ill Hospitalized Patients: The Study to Understand Prognoses and Preferences for Outcomes and Risks of Treatment (SUPPORT)," *Journal of the American Medical Association* 274 (1995): 1591–1598; and L. Snyder and A. L. Caplan, "Die Hard: End-of-Life Care in America," *Pennsylvania Medicine* 99 (1996): 10–11.

12. D. Humphry, *Lawful Exit: The Limits of Freedom for Help in Dying* (Sarasota, Fla.: Norris Lane Press, 1993); and Battin, *The Least Worst Death.*

13. M. A. Drickamer, M. A. Lee, and L. Ganzini, "Practical Issues in Physician Assisted Suicide," *Annals of Internal Medicine* 126 (1997): 146–151.

14. S. W. Tolle, "Care of the Dying: Clinical and Financial Lessons from the Oregon Experience," *Annals of Internal Medicine* 128 (1998): 567–568.

15. Task Force to Improve the Care of Terminally Ill Oregonians, *The Oregon Death with Dignity Act: A Guidebook for Health Care Providers* (Portland: Oregon Health Sciences University, 1998).

16. F. G. Miller et al., "Regulating Physician-Assisted Death," *New England Journal of Medicine* 331 (1994): 119–123; and C. H. Baron et al., "A Model State Act to Authorize and Regulate Physician-Assisted Suicide," *Harvard Journal on Legislation* 33 (1996): 1–34.

17. S. Heilig et al., "Physician-Hastened Death: Advisory Guidelines for the San Francisco Bay Area from the Bay Area Network of Ethics Committees," *Western Journal of Medicine* 166 (1997): 370–378.

18. C. H. Coleman and A. R. Fleischman, "Guidelines for Physician-Assisted Suicide: Can the Challenge Be Met?" *Journal of Law, Medicine, and Ethics* 24 (1996): 217–224.

19. Ibid.; and Smith, *Forced Exit.*

20. Coleman and Fleischman, "Guidelines for Physician-Assisted Suicide"; D. Callahan and M. White, "The Legalization of Physician-Assisted Suicide: Creating a Regulatory Potemkin Village," *University of Richmond Law Review* 30 (1996): 1–83; and F. G. Miller, "A Communitarian Approach to Physician-Assisted Death," *Cambridge Quarterly of Healthcare Ethics* 6 (1997): 78–87.

21. G. A. Larue, *Playing God: Fifty Religions' Views on Your Right to Die* (Wakefield, R.I.: Moyer Bell, 1996).

22. Task Force, *The Oregon Death with Dignity Act.*

23. I. Byock, *Dying Well: Peace and Possibilities at the End of Life* (New York: Riverhead Books, 1997); M. S. Peck, *Denial of the Soul: Spiritual and Medical Perspectives on Euthanasia and Mortality* (New York: Random House, 1997); M. Albom, *Tuesdays with Morrie: An Old Man, a Young Man, and Life's Greatest Lesson* (New York: Doubleday, 1997); M. Webb, *The Good Death: The New American Search to Reshape the End of Life* (New York: Bantam, 1997); E. Kubler-Ross, *The Wheel of Life: A Memoir of Living and Dying* (New York: Scribner, 1997); P. McNees, *Dying: A Book of Comfort* (New York: Warner, 1998); and M. Vitez, *Final Choices: Seeking the Good Death* (Philadelphia: Camino, 1998).

24. Nuland, *How We Die;* and Vitez, *Final Choices.*

25. T. E. Quill, C. K. Cassel, and D. E. Meier, "Care of the Hopelessly Ill: Proposed Clinical Criteria for Physician-Assisted Suicide," *New England Journal of Medicine* 327 (1992); 1380–1384.

26. Miller et al., "Regulating Physician-Assisted Death"; Baron et al., "A Model State Act to Authorize and Regulate Physician-Assisted Suicide"; and Heilig et al., "Physician-Hastened Death."

27. E. W. Young et al., "Report of the Northern California Conference for Guidelines on Aid-in-Dying: Definitions, Differences, Convergences, Conclusions," *Western Journal of Medicine* 166 (1997): 381–388.

28. Task Force, *The Oregon Death with Dignity Act.*

29. New York State Task Force on Life and the Law, *When Death Is Sought: Assisted Suicide and Euthanasia in the Medical Context* (New York: Task Force on Life and the Law, 1994).

30. Callahan and White, "The Legalization of Physician-Assisted Suicide."

31. Tolle, "Care of the Dying."

32. Task Force, *The Oregon Death with Dignity Act.*

33. Sneiderman, "Euthanasia in the Netherlands"; and J. J. Fins, "Physician-Assisted Suicide and the Right to Care," *Cancer Control* 3 (1996): 272–278.

34. Albom, *Tuesdays with Morrie*; Vitez, *Final Choices*; and D. Rabe, *A Question of Mercy* (New York: Grove, 1998).

35. V. P. Tilden and M. A. Lee, "Oregon's Physician-Assisted Suicide Legislation: Troubling Issues for Families," *Journal of Family Nursing* 3 (1997): 120–129.

36. Albom, *Tuesdays with Morrie*; Webb, *The Good Death*; P. Anderson, *All of Us: Americans Talk about the Meaning of Death* (New York: Delacorte, 1996); T. E. Quill, *A Midwife through the Dying Process: Stories of Healing and Hard Choices at the End of Life* (Baltimore: Johns Hopkins University Press, 1996); and E. J. Emanuel and L. L. Emanuel, "The Promise of a Good Death," *Lancet* 351, Supplement 2 (1998): 21–29.

37. SUPPORT Principal Investigators, "A Controlled Trial to Improve Care for Seriously Ill Hospitalized Patients"; and M. J. Field and C. K. Cassel, eds., *Approaching Death: Improving Care at the End of Life* (Washington: National Academy Press, 1997).

38. A. E. Chin et al., "Legalized Physician-Assisted Suicide in Oregon— The First Year's Experience," *New England Journal of Medicine* 340 (1999): 577–583.

39. Sneiderman, "Euthanasia in the Netherlands"; Miller, "A Communitarian Approach to Physician-Assisted Death"; and Vitez, *Final Choices.*

Four

KATHY FABER-LANGENDOEN, M.D., AND JASON H. T. KARLAWISH, M.D.

Ought Assisted Suicide Be Only Physician *Assisted?*

MULTIPLE PUBLIC AND PROFESSIONAL opinion polls, and implementation of the Oregon Death with Dignity Act, show that legal assisted suicide for competent terminally ill persons is gaining acceptance in this country.[1] Numerous failed attempts to convict Jack Kevorkian for assisting with suicide suggest the lack of public sympathy for enforcing laws prohibiting assisted suicide, although this sentiment does not extend to euthanasia, for which Kevorkian was convicted of murder.

In discussions in the media, courts, legislatures, and professional societies, assistance with suicide is generally assumed to be a physician task: It is called "physician-assisted suicide." All legislative attempts, Oregon's law, public referenda, and proposed guidelines focus on physicians' responsibilities and procedures in helping patients end their lives.[2]

However, deep, principled division exists within the medical profession as to whether physician-assisted suicide violates professional integrity.[3] Concerns are also raised that patients may not have access to physicians with adequate training, certification, or professional support to take the lead in assisted suicide. Among the twenty-three Oregon patients who received prescriptions for lethal medications in 1998, six consulted multiple physicians before successfully obtaining the prescription.[4] Equally important to the issue of access is whether physicians are in fact the best professionals to take the lead. Physician qualifications in end-of-life care are not unique or even exemplary.[5] If society wants access to competent and effective assisted suicide, it ought to consider to what extent other professions are better equipped to assist. Key questions include the following: Ought assisted suicide be only "physician-assisted suicide?" Could and should another health care profession replace physicians? For example, why not have "nurse-assisted suicide?" Or could a variety of interested health care professionals take on this task?

The point of these questions is not to advance an argument either for or against assisted suicide. Alternatives to assisted suicide exist, including maximal efforts at palliative care, terminal sedation, and refusal of food and fluids, and are thought by many to be more morally acceptable. However, some find these alternatives inadequate, and Oregonians were sufficiently persuaded to have twice voted to legalize physician-assisted suicide. While the debate about the morality of legalizing assisted suicide continues, both opponents and proponents have an interest in ensuring that the practice is appropriately restricted, analogous to the public policy debates about abortion since *Roe v. Wade.* The aim of this paper is to define both the necessity and the limits of the physician's role in assisted suicide by asking the question: Ought assisted suicide be only *physician* assisted? At heart, our argument is not about the ethics of *whether* to do assisted suicide but, given the legal option, the ethics of *how* to do it. Our premise is that health care professionals ought not act outside their spheres of professional competence.

This chapter examines the tasks inherent within assisted suicide and the competence of various people who might be able to do them. The current predominance of a physician role in assisted suicide may be misdirected, misleading, and even unnecessary. While physician involvement is necessary, we argue it is not sufficient to assure that patients requesting assisted suicide receive the best care. We will show this by examining the nature of assisting a suicide and potential roles of nonphysician health professionals in assisting suicide.

The Nature of Assisting a Suicide

In most proposed guidelines and regulations for assisted suicide, physicians have key roles. In contrast, other health care professionals either are not mentioned or are involved at the physician's discretion.[6] Physicians are expected to communicate prognostic information, provide palliative care options, assess depression, and provide the patients with the means to commit suicide. Although a physician's skills are necessary for some of these tasks (such as communicating prognostic information), medical means are not necessary for a person to end his or her life.

Suicide is possible using a variety of nonmedical methods such as guns, carbon monoxide, and asphyxiation.[7] Unfortunately, these methods can be violent, messy, variably effective, socially isolating, or repugnant. In addition, a person could voluntarily decide to stop eating and drinking, dying by means of dehydration (a method that, while probably legal, is also morally controversial).[8] This process, however, takes a great deal of resolve on the part of the patient and caregivers and may take several days to weeks. The use of lethal doses of prescription medications has been advocated because it is quick; appears to be more humane, effective, and peaceful; and allows the person to die in the presence of loved ones.

The tendency to medicalize assisted suicide as a last resort for competent terminally ill patients bears more than a passing resemblance to the medicalization of capital punishment in the last half of this century (from hanging and firing squad to lethal injection). Physicians appear to be the most efficient and skilled profession to effectively and humanely end a life. As is the case with capital punishment, physician expertise may be called upon in two areas: the process of assessment prior to ending a life, and the provision or administration of the means.[9] While physicians play key roles in the assessment process (evaluating prognosis, providing palliative care options, and assessing depression), the provision of medical means *per se*, as has been the case with capital punishment, need not be done only by physicians, should physicians judge that assisting suicide is incompatible with professional values.[10]

Moreover, even if assisted suicide were accepted as a medical task, physicians may not be the only or even the best profession to implement humane and effective assisted suicide. The physician's skills in this area might even be surpassed by other health care professionals. In light of the medical profession's ambivalence about accepting this role, the predominant role physicians have been assigned needs careful scrutiny.

Potential Roles of Physicians and Nonphysicians in Assisted Suicide

As society legalizes assisted suicide, it maintains interests in confining it to appropriate cases, using methods that are effective but neither unaesthetic nor violent, and protecting patients and families' privacy. To meet these interests, we suggest that assisted suicide by prescription of lethal medication requires, at minimum, the following steps:

1. Assessment of the request for assisted suicide
2. Preparing the person for dying
3. Providing the means
4. Providing support as requested during administration of the medications and the person's dying
5. Managing complications
6. Reporting the assisted suicide
7. Overall coordination and oversight

Examining the competency of various kinds of people who might have a role in the individual's assisted suicide shows that these seven steps are not the exclusive domain of physicians.

1. ASSESSMENT OF THE REQUEST FOR ASSISTED SUICIDE

The initial assessment of requests for assisted suicide is clearly within the physician's expertise. Physicians generally assume primary responsibility for communicating information about diagnosis, prognosis, and the full range of treatment options; ensuring that every reasonable attempt to provide palliative care has been made; and assessing concomitant factors (such as depression) that may adversely influence a patient's decision making. The task of assessing requests for assisted suicide is an effort to help patients consider all other alternatives, often with the hope that they will find an option other than suicide to be acceptable.[11]

While some might argue that even this degree of involvement entails an unacceptable level of moral complicity with an intended suicide, we believe that the physician's role here is analogous to that of the psychiatrist opposed to the death penalty who is called upon to offer an opinion as to whether the accused is mentally fit to stand trial for a capital offense or the physician consulted by the Social Security Administration to provide a medical assessment of whether a patient is too disabled to work. The physician contributes important information about the patient's diagnosis, prognosis, and response to treatments, but others decide that the patient is incompetent or disabled and act upon the consequences of that decision. Assessment of a request need not imply moral agreement with the final outcome, be it the death penalty, disability determination, or assisted suicide.

2. PREPARING THE PERSON FOR DYING

Other critically important tasks are far outside physician expertise and are best accomplished through the expertise of others.[12] For many patients, spiritual issues are a part of confronting death,[13] and contemplating suicide raises spiritual questions of control, the meaning of suf-

fering, and final destiny. Insofar as spiritual concerns translate into religious beliefs for many Americans, physicians are often ill equipped to
deal with such issues, being less religious, less likely to believe in God,
and less likely to believe in prayer than the general population.[14] In
addition, patients choosing assisted suicide merit maximal efforts at
relieving physical and mental distress. Experience in hospice shows that
skilled nurses effectively provide this care with physician support. Finally, there is the need to assess whether potential coercive factors are
unduly influencing the person's request. Factors such as family dynam-
ics and economic pressures are best confronted by those expert in the
psychosocial aspects of care. Addressing issues of coercion, spiritual
concerns, and symptom control clearly requires expertise beyond that
of physicians and is often better provided by nurses, social workers, and
clergy or other spiritual advisers. Physician involvement alone is insufficient.

3. PROVIDING THE MEANS

Public and legislative debates continue to focus on the task of prescribing lethal drugs for assisted suicide,[15] and state regulations now grant
physicians exclusive prescribing authority for medications commonly
used for assisted suicide. Although nurses and physician assistants are
generally prohibited from prescribing schedule II drugs such as seco-
barbital or morphine, many states already grant limited independent
prescribing authority to nonphysician health care professionals, including physician assistants and advanced practice nurses.[16] Physicians need
not be the only ones who can prescribe drugs commonly used for
assisted suicide. Nurse practitioners or physician assistants could be
granted independent prescription authority to exercise after a physician certifies that a patient meets the prognostic and diagnostic criteria
for assisted suicide and is competent to make the decision to commit
suicide. Expanding prescribing authority may improve access to assisted suicide if too few physicians are willing to assist.[17] However, giving
nonphysicians independent prescribing authority opens up the possibility that the process of assisted suicide could be short-circuited without physician involvement, a risk that may be unacceptable given the
necessity of their involvement in assessing diagnosis, prognosis, and the
full range of care options.

4. PROVIDING SUPPORT AS REQUESTED DURING ADMINISTRATION OF THE MEDICATIONS AND THE PATIENT'S DYING

One of the arguments advanced for legalizing assisted suicide is that
legalization allows people to die in the presence of people who care for
them, without fear of putting these people at risk of prosecution. Pa-

tients and families may choose to have others present to lend emotional support and monitor the dying process. Such assistance could be provided by a variety of professionals, including nurses, physicians, social workers, and clergy. While a physician ought to be available should complications arise, the physician is unlikely to be the key player in attending to the patient's and family's needs during the dying process.

5. MANAGING COMPLICATIONS

The problem of how to manage a failed suicide attempt presents a task unlike any previously assumed by health care professionals. When suicide is intended but the patient does not die, who should take further steps, if any, to end the person's life? While physicians again clearly have the medical means to end life under these circumstances, there is likely to be even greater professional resistance to this than to prescribing lethal drugs for self-administration.

Exact data on the incidence of this problem is difficult to obtain, given the illegality of assisted suicide in most jurisdictions. Anecdotes exist of assisted suicides gone awry, with patients either vomiting the drugs or the doses being insufficient, so that family members or others eventually ended the person's life by asphyxiation with a pillow or plastic bag.[18] One could argue that these cases result from "amateur" attempts and that such events are far less likely to occur in the hands of properly trained experts. While the Dutch practice in ending patients' lives generally proceeds by the use of intravenous sedation followed by intravenous paralytics (and thus fall under the category of euthanasia), some Dutch data about the use of oral drugs (applicable to assisted suicide) are available.[19] If sufficient quantities of barbiturates are ingested without vomiting, most patients die within one hour; approximately 25 percent survive up to five hours, with occasional survivors up to twenty-four hours. Of seventy-five reported cases using oral medications, 77 percent of patients died without further intervention. However, 20 percent died only after additional administration of intravenous paralytics, suggesting that oral medication alone may be either insufficient or unacceptably slow for a substantial minority of patients wishing to end their lives.[20] These data suggest that failed attempts happen.

Although dealing with failed attempts at suicide fall far outside the physician's traditional duty, someone (whether physician, family, nurse, or others) will have to attend to such events. Regulations that do not anticipate this outcome and specify who will take action are shortsighted and will not serve patients well. Expanding the capacity and authority to complete failed attempts to other competent and willing health care professionals may protect patients' ability to have their lives ended humanely but will extend medical practice from assisted suicide to euthanasia, an extension that many will find unacceptable.

6. REPORTING THE ASSISTED SUICIDE

In Oregon and most guidelines, completed assisted suicides must be reported. This step is of little importance to the individual, but it serves important ends for the public, health care professionals, and future people who seek assisted suicide, providing a way to monitor practice. Although it cannot correct missteps in a particular suicide, it can help assure assisted suicide for future people meets established procedural safeguards. In general, physicians report death by completing death certificates. This practice leads one to assume that physicians should also be the one to report an assisted suicide, as the Oregon law stipulates. But if other professionals play key roles in the steps that lead up to an assisted suicide, they too ought to report their involvement in an assisted suicide. Perhaps the most sensible model for reporting is that all professionals who participated in the assisted suicide should jointly report it. This broad documentation serves to assure the public that patients receive the best possible multidisciplinary care and that all professionals who participate account for their role.

7. OVERALL COORDINATION AND OVERSIGHT

Assisted suicide requires a sequence of complex and important tasks. Rarely will a single health care professional be expert in all of these tasks, and several of the essential components can and perhaps should be done by professionals other than physicians. However, the Oregon Death with Dignity Act assigns physicians this role of overall oversight and coordination. This likely reflects the traditional lead of physicians in orchestrating medical care, particularly in the diagnosis or treatment of disease. But assisted suicide involves tasks and skills that extend beyond the physician's abilities. Even in areas that do fall under the physician's domain, such as pain and symptom management, actual practice is often shamefully inadequate.[21]

If no single health care profession has all of the skills needed, perhaps the best model is multidisciplinary care such as practiced in rehabilitation and hospice. When patients die under the care of hospice, it is often the hospice nurse who coordinates the care and ensures that emotional, financial, relational, and medical issues are each given their due, while physicians retain key roles in prescribing and, at times, compassionate support to the patient and family. The traditional hierarchies of authority within the health care professions as well as physician-oriented methods of reimbursement might make the orchestration of assisted suicide seem to be a physician-led task. But this responsibility could just as well be assigned to a nurse or other health care professional. It could even be extended to someone outside the health care professions, such as clergy. The model of another professional serving to oversee and coordinate an assisted suicide might have a physician assessing the request and a multidisciplinary team led by a nurse performing the other steps. Although this team could include a physician, it need not be led by one.

Whether this model would better ensure that the multiple facets of a request for assisted suicide were attended to is unknown, but it is a matter that could be subjected to empirical scrutiny, much as the Dutch have examined their practices of assisted suicide and euthanasia. On a principled level, having other professionals oversee the process of assisted suicide both emphasizes the critical participation of nonphysician health care professionals and recognizes the physician's limited expertise in the various tasks involved.

Discussion

The debate over assisted suicide is overly focused on the physician's role. Assisted suicide requires physician involvement, but physicians' limited competence in performing the full range of tasks, the competencies of other professions, and the possibility that other professions could expand their authority in this area suggest that *physician-*assisted suicide is a far too narrow a construct of the task. The need for a multidisciplinary approach to assisted suicide is precisely the same need that led to the formation of hospice programs to attend to the dying and their families, a model that may be applicable to assisted suicide. The federal government, through Medicare regulations, will certify only hospices that provide physician, nursing, social work, and spiritual services. Regulations for assisted suicide could also be written to ensure that those seeking assisted suicide have access to a skilled and multidisciplinary group of experts. A physician may need to be part of, but not necessarily the leader of, that group.

Statements from nonphysician health care professional organizations demonstrate that other health care professionals face the same ambivalence as physicians and are still defining their willingness to associate their professions with assisted suicide. The American Nurses Association and the Oncology Nursing Society have published statements against assisted suicide; the Oregon State Nurses' Association has an ambivalent statement regarding nurse involvement.[22] The American Association of Physician Assistants has an ambiguous statement regarding physician assistant involvement, although it does state that physician assistants may act if they are following a doctor's orders.[23] Social workers are encouraged by the National Association of Social Workers to explore alternatives to assisted suicide with patients. That association states that social workers ought to be free to be present for patients and families during an assisted suicide, although the policy cautions social workers against assisting with administration of lethal medications, adding that "it is inappropriate for social workers to . . . personally participate in the commission of an act of assisted suicide."[24] The 1994 Code of Ethics of the American Pharmacists Association does not directly address physician-assisted suicide. Recent surveys show that approximately half of pharmacists support physicians' or other health care professionals' assisting in suicide and that a sizeable minority would agree to dispense drugs for this purpose.[25]

The range of opinion regarding the ethics and morality of assisted suicide suggests that no health care profession is likely to unequivocally embrace the provision of lethal medications for assisted suicide as part of its profession or to take the lead in coordinating the care of patients wishing to end their lives. However, that same ambivalence and variation in opinion suggests that sufficient support may exist for developing a new health care structure (analogous to hospice) derived from multiple health care disciplines that is willing to provide assistance. This new structure, which could include physicians, nurses, clergy, social workers, and pharmacists, would be united by the common goal of defining the standards and training required to fulfill an individual's request for assisted suicide. State laws and regulations could be rewritten to grant this multidisciplinary structure the authority to provide assisted suicide.

Conclusion

Stipulating that assisted suicide be *physician*-assisted may assure society a level of review and exploration of alternatives that may not occur where assisted suicide remains a private, illegal act. But physician-assisted suicide is far too narrow a construct to meet the public's expectation that some individuals ought to have access to humane and effective assisted suicide. Physician assistance, while perhaps necessary, is insufficient to ensure that assisted suicide is restricted to appropriate cases and occurs in an appropriate manner. This is likely to be especially true if assisted suicide becomes more widely legal: The average physician is arguably ill prepared to lead assisted suicide. The willingness of other health care professionals, including nurses, social workers, and clergy, to participate and even take the lead in assisting suicides is critical to meeting society's interest that assisted suicide, if available, is humane, effective, and confined to appropriate cases. As long as legislation and guidelines focus exclusively on the physician's role, our laws and regulations will fall short of meeting this assurance.

REFERENCES

1. M. Angell, "The Supreme Court and Physician-Assisted Suicide: The Ultimate Right," *New England Journal of Medicine* 336 (1997): 50–53; J. G. Bachman et al., "Attitudes of Michigan Physicians and the Public toward Legalizing Physician-Assisted Suicide and Voluntary Euthanasia," *New England Journal of Medicine* 334 (1996); 303–315; H. Brody, "Assisted Death: A Compassionate Response to a Medical Failure," *New England Journal of Medicine* 327 (1992): 1384–1388; J. S. Cohen et al., "Attitudes toward Assisted Suicide and Euthanasia among Physicians in Washington State," *New England Journal of Medicine* 331 (1994): 89–94; D. Doukas et al., "Attitudes and Behaviors on Physician-Assisted Death: A Study of Michigan Oncologists," *Journal of Clinical Oncology* 13 (1995): 1055–1061; E. Emanuel, "Euthanasia and Physician-Assisted Suicide: Attitudes and Experiences of Oncology Patients, Oncologists, and the Public," *Lancet* 347 (1996): 1805–1810; M. E. Suarez-Almazar, M. Belzile, and E. Bruera, "Euthanasia and Physician-Assisted Suicide: A Comparable Survey of Physicians, Terminally Ill Cancer Patients, and the General Population," *Journal of Clinical Oncology* 15 (1997): 418–427; and M. Gillespie, "Kevorkian to Face Murder Charges," Gallup Poll Releases, 19 March 1999, <www.gallup.com/poll/releases/pr990319.asp> (29 November 2000).
2. A. L. Caplan, L. Snyder, and K. Faber-Langendoen, "The Role of Guidelines in the Practice of Physician-Assisted Suicide," *Annals of Internal Medicine* 132 (2000): 476–481.
3. D. Callahan, "Self-Extinction: The Morality of the Helping Hand," in *Physician-Assisted Suicide*, ed. R. F. Weir (Indianapolis: Indiana University Press, 1997), 69–85; I. Byock, "Physician-Assisted Suicide Is Not an Acceptable Practice for Physicians," in *Physician-Assisted Suicide*, 107–135; and H. Brody, "Assisting in Patient Suicides Is an Acceptable Practice for Physicians," in *Physician-Assisted Suicide*, 136–151.
4. A. E. Chin et al., "Legalized Physician-Assisted Suicide in Oregon—The First Year's Experience," *New England Journal of Medicine* 340 (1999): 577–583.
5. M. J. Field and C. K. Cassel, eds., *Approaching Death: Improving Care at the End of Life* (Washington: National Academy Press, 1997), 363–382; and C. Cleeland et al., "Pain and Its Treatment in Outpatients with Metastatic Cancer," *New England Journal of Medicine* 330 (1994): 592–596.
6. Caplan, Snyder, and Faber-Langendoen, "The Role of Guidelines in the Practice of Physician-Assisted Suicide."
7. D. Humphry, *Final Exit: The Practicalities of Self-Deliverance and Assisted Suicide for the Dying* (Secaucus, N.J.: Hemlock Society, 1991).
8. F. G. Miller and D. E. Meier, "Voluntary Death: A Comparison of Terminal Dehydration and Physician-Assisted Suicide," *Annals of Internal Medicine* 128 (1998): 559–562.
9. E. H. Loewy, "Healing and Killing, Harming and Not Harming: Physician Participation in Euthanasia and Capital Punishment," *Journal of Clinical Ethics* 3 (1992): 29–34.
10. Council on Ethical and Judicial Affairs, American Medical Association,

"Physician Participation in Capital Punishment," *Journal of the American Medical Association* 270 (1993): 365–368.

11. J. A. Tulsky, R. Ciampa, and E. J. Rosen, "Responding to Legal Requests for Physician-Assisted Suicide," *Annals of Internal Medicine* 132 (2000): 494–499.

12. S. H. Miles, "Physician-Assisted Suicide and the Profession's Gyrocompass," *Hastings Center Report* 25 (1995): 17–19.

13. Nathan Cummings Foundation and Fetzer Institute, *Spiritual Beliefs and the Dying Process* (New York: Nathan Cummings Foundation, October 1997).

14. L. M. Goldfarb et al., "Medical Student and Patient Attitudes toward Religion and Spirituality in the Recovery Process," *American Journal of Drug and Alcohol Abuse* 22 (1996): 549–561; T. A. Maugans and W. C. Wadland, "Religion and Family Medicine: A Survey of Physicians and Patients," *Journal of Family Practice* 32 (1991): 210–213; J. Neeleman and M. B. King, "Psychiatrists' Religious Attitudes in Relation to Their Clinical Practice: A Survey of 231 Psychiatrists," *Acta Psychiatrica Scandinavica* 88 (1993): 420–424; and H. G. Koenig et al., "Religious Perspectives of Doctors, Nurses, Patients, and Families," *Journal of Pastoral Care* 45 (1991): 254–267.

15. *Lethal Drug Abuse Prevention Act of 1998*, H.R. 4006, 105th Cong., 2d Sess. (1998).

16. National Association of Boards of Pharmacy, *1997–98 Survey of Pharmacy Law* (Park Ridge, Ill.: NABP, 1997), 65–73.

17. Chin et al., "Legalized Physician-Assisted Suicide in Oregon."

18. S. Jamison, *Final Acts of Love* (New York: G. P. Putnam's Sons, 1995).

19. G. van der Wal et al., "The Use of Drugs for Euthanasia and Assisted Suicide in Family Practice" (in Dutch), *Nederlands Tijdschrift voor Geneeskunde* 136 (1992): 1299–1305; and P. V. Admiraal, "Toepassing van euthanatica," *Nederlands Tijdschrift voor Geneeskunde* 139 (1995): 265–268.

20. Ibid.

21. Cleeland et al., "Pain and Its Treatment in Outpatients with Metastatic Cancer."

22. American Nurses Association, "Position Statement on Assisted Suicide" (Washington: ANA, 1994), 1–10; Oncology Nursing Society, "The Oncology Nursing Society's Endorsement of the American Nurses Association Position Statements on Active Euthanasia and Assisted Suicide" (Pittsburgh: ONS, 1995); and "ONA Provides Guidance on Nurses' Dilemma," *Oregon Nursing* 62 (1997): 5.

23. M. P. Battin and A. Lipman, eds., *Drug Use in Assisted Suicide and Euthanasia* (New York: Haworth Press, 1996), 267–272.

24. National Association of Social Workers, "Client Self-Determination in End-of-Life Decisions: A Statement of the National Association of Social Workers," *Social Work Speaks: NASW Policy Statements*, 3d ed. (Washington: NASW Press, 1994), 58–61.

25. M. T. Rupp and H. L. Isenhower, "Pharmacists' Attitudes toward Physician-Assisted Suicide," *American Journal of Hospital Pharmacy* 51 (1994): 69–74.

Five

DAVID ORENTLICHER, M.D., J.D., AND LOIS SNYDER, J.D.

Can Assisted Suicide Be Regulated?

IN THIS CHAPTER WE CONSIDER important questions about whether and how a legal right to assisted suicide can be regulated. We do not re-open the debate about whether assisted suicide, particularly physician-assisted suicide, should or should not be widely available—although, of course, the stringency of regulation does affect how widely available such a right would be. Instead, assuming there are times when assisted suicide is morally acceptable in theory, it will address whether a right to assisted suicide that is morally safe can be implemented in practice. That is, can regulations for assisted suicide that will truly prevent serious abuse be designed? Or are the difficulties with regulation so severe that it is preferable for patients to rely on the alternatives to suicide that are currently permitted (e.g., terminal sedation or the refusal of food and water)? Can useful analogies be made to regulation in other contexts?

Other chapters in this book[1] address the distinction between assisted suicide and treatment withdrawal and the question of whether assisted suicide should be *physician*-assisted suicide. Those issues are not revisited here.

Background Considerations

Regulations serve several important goals. Most importantly, they provide guidance as to the line between permissible and impermissible behavior. We permit people to drive at some speeds but not at other speeds. Similarly, assisted-suicide regulations typically would limit the practice to *physician*-assisted suicide and to patients who possess decision-making capacity.

When lines are drawn between the permissible and the impermissible, and mechanisms implemented to enforce those lines, public trust can be enhanced. Society will tolerate potentially dangerous practices only if there are adequate protections against the risk of harm. Moreover, many individuals will be willing to make their behavior conform to what is morally and legally required only if they are assured that others will do the same. Well-enforced regulations can help provide that assurance.

Regulations also serve an important monitoring function. As new regulations are implemented, data can be collected and analyzed to see if the regulations are working as intended or whether modifications are necessary to ensure more appropriate behavior.

Regulations have drawbacks as well as benefits. They can be cumbersome and administratively inefficient. They can also be counterproductive. For example, procedural requirements for the withdrawal of life-sustaining treatment from incompetent patients prevent premature withdrawals from patients who would want treatment continued. However, they also can interfere with the rights of other patients who would want treatment withdrawn. If a state requires clear and convincing evidence of patient's wishes, and the wishes must have specifically anticipated the patient's current condition, patients may be treated against what would have likely been their preferences.[2]

Because regulations have advantages and disadvantages, it is often difficult to decide exactly how much regulation is appropriate. If regulation is too light, serious harms can result. If regulation is too heavy, different harms can result. Too permissive a right to assisted suicide might lead to many premature deaths. Too restrictive a right (or no right) might result in unnecessary suffering.

Arguments about Regulatability

Key questions, then, are whether assisted suicide can be permitted under certain conditions and, if so, under which conditions? Even if we consider assisted suicide to be morally permissible in some situations, it might not be possible to permit the practice for the morally permissible cases without also ending up with assisted suicide for morally impermissible cases.

1. *Is it possible to legalize assisted suicide in some circumstances without ultimately opening the door to assisted suicide and/or euthanasia for all indi-*

viduals? Proposals for assisted suicide typically permit only physicians to assist, and they generally would not permit euthanasia. Proposals also limit the right to patients who are terminally ill and who have the mental capacity to make medical decisions. For example, all four limitations are part of the Oregon Death with Dignity Act, the only law in the United States permitting physician-assisted suicide. Under that law, patients must be competent adults and within six months of death to exercise their statutory rights. The right granted is a right of the patient to obtain a "prescription for medication to end his or her life in a humane and dignified manner."

As many commentators have observed, however, it is difficult in practice—and in principle—to distinguish between patients who are terminally ill and those who are not terminally ill.[3] For patients with solid tumors, predictions of life expectancy are reasonably good. For patients with congestive heart failure, however, it is not possible to predict with much certainty whether they can live for only a few months or another year or two.[4] Moreover, even when we can make reliable determinations of life expectancy, it does not follow that the patient's right to die should hinge on whether the patient is terminally ill. If a patient has an incurable disease and is suffering greatly, should it matter whether the patient has five months to live or twenty-five months to live? Indeed, it can be argued that the patient who has twenty-five months to live will experience much more total suffering than the patient with only five months to live.[5]

Similarly, it may be difficult to hold the line between assisted suicide and euthanasia. Many dying patients will be too disabled to take the lethal dose of medication, but their desire to die may be just as justified as that of patients who retain the ability to commit suicide. Arguably, it is unfair and discriminatory to permit less disabled patients the option to end their lives while denying that option to more disabled persons. Finally, some argue, it should not matter whether the patient is competent.[6] If the patient left explicit instructions for euthanasia in the event of incompetence and serious illness, why shouldn't those instructions be carried out as would other instructions left by the patient?[7]

Experience supports concern that a limited right to assisted suicide will lead to an unlimited right to both assisted suicide and euthanasia. The history of the right to refuse life-sustaining treatment is a history of discarded distinctions. Whether the patient is terminally ill, whether the treatment is a ventilator or a feeding tube, or whether the treatment is withheld or withdrawn are no longer considered conceptual restrictions to the right to refuse treatment.[8]

These arguments are well taken, but there are important counter-arguments. First, the concern about expansions beyond a limited right to assisted suicide assumes that such expansions would be wrong. However, good moral reasons may exist to support a right to assisted suicide for some patients who are not terminally ill or a right to euthanasia for some patients who are unable to take medications by themselves. Indeed, it may be more troublesome to withhold life-sustaining treatment from a "pleasantly senile" patient who had never expressed treatment preferences than to permit euthanasia for a competent patient who is within a few days of death and who is suffering greatly. But if expansions of a right to assisted suicide would involve practices that are not morally different from assisted suicide for the terminally ill, it is hard to see why expansions of the right would be unacceptable. If society decides that assisted suicide for the terminally ill is morally appropriate, it would not be wrong to also permit assisted suicide for other patients who have the same moral justification for ending their lives that terminally ill patients have. If, on the other hand, there are important moral differences between assisted suicide and euthanasia or between suicide for the terminally ill and suicide for those who are not terminally ill, those differences ought to provide sufficient protection against the risk of expansion. The right to abortion has not led to a right to infanticide or even to a right to abortion after viability, in large part because there are important moral differences between pre-viable fetuses and viable fetuses or infants.

Second, the expansion of the right to refuse life-sustaining treatment has been greatly overstated by many commentators. Although it is true in theory that the patient's diagnosis and prognosis are no longer relevant for purposes of treatment withdrawal, in practice they matter very much. As illustrated by court decisions in Michigan, New Jersey, and Wisconsin, legal standards make it much more difficult to withdraw treatment from incompetent patients who are neither terminally ill nor permanently unconscious.[9]

Third, in terms of the reasons for the legal distinction between assisted suicide and treatment withdrawal, there is good reason to think that a right to assisted suicide for the terminally ill would remain limited. It has been argued that the distinction between assisted suicide and treatment withdrawal has existed not because of any real moral difference between the two acts, but because the distinction does a generally good job of sorting morally justified from morally unjustified patient deaths.[10] In this view, the morality of a patient's death depends on the patient's condition, not on the mechanism of the patient's death. That is, the right to refuse life-sustaining treatment ultimately rests on the moral sentiment that people should be able to die when they are suffering greatly from an irreversible illness, rather than on the position that patients have an autonomy right to refuse any and all bodily invasions. In this view, we allow treatment withdrawal but deny assisted suicide because the *typical* person who refuses life-sustaining treatment is irreversibly ill and suffering greatly (and therefore morally justified in wanting to die) while the *typical* person who wishes to commit suicide is not irreversibly ill (and therefore not morally justified in wanting to die).[11] Permitting assisted suicide but limiting the right to the terminally ill may enable the law to better sort morally justified from morally unjustified deaths. Accordingly, further expansions of the right would occur only if necessary to better serve the goal of sorting morally justified from morally unjustified patient deaths.

2. *Even if lines can be drawn, are the lines likely to be observed?* As mentioned, many proposals would limit physician-assisted suicide to terminally ill patients. But it is not always clear when a patient becomes terminally ill. Similarly, although a law might require that the patient be competent and not suffering from treatable depression, physicians are often not very good at detecting treatable depression in their patients.[12] Requirements of second opinions are not a foolproof safeguard. Physicians can often find sympathetic colleagues who will ratify their opinions.

Without doubt, there would be slippage. Even with the most careful guidelines and the most stringent safeguards, mistakes will be made. However, that is not necessarily the correct measure of success or failure. Rather, it may be more appropriate to ask whether the mistakes would be any more frequent or more serious with assisted suicide than with treatment withdrawal. Patients often refuse life-sustaining treatment because they believe they are terminally ill or irreversibly dependent on life-sustaining treatment. Medical uncertainty means that many of these patients might choose death on the basis of an erroneous assumption about their prognosis, just as patients might choose assisted suicide in the mistaken belief that they are terminally ill. Concerns about treatable depression are also an issue for treatment withdrawal. Patients who refuse a ventilator, dialysis, or other treatments may have an undetected depression.

Commentators often cite the Dutch experience to show that slippage is inevitable.[13] Leading studies have found that in about 25–30 percent of cases involving euthanasia or assisted suicide, patients did not make an explicit and contemporaneous request to have their life ended, as required under the safeguards developed by the medical profession and the courts in the Netherlands.[14] However, these and other rule violations need not reflect the administration of euthanasia against the patient's wishes or in response to coercion by family members or physicians. Although that does happen, the violations often reflect two types of deviation: (1) failures to adhere to reporting requirements or to obtain outside review[15] and (2) situations in which euthanasia is probably consistent with the patient's wishes but in which the evidence of the patient's wishes does not meet the formal requirement of contemporaneous, consistent, and persistent expressions.[16] In other words, the abuses in the Netherlands often involve violations of the letter but not the spirit of the law.

Still, there may be undetected abuses in the Netherlands. In most cases of physician-assisted suicide or euthanasia, physicians do not meet their legal obligation to report the case to public authorities. But even if we accept the most serious charges of abuse regarding the Netherlands' experience, it still does not follow that we can distinguish between physician-assisted suicide and withdrawal of life-sustaining treatment. The Netherlands experience may show that legalizing euthanasia or assisted suicide leads to abuse, but the same concerns of abuse arise with the withdrawal of life-sustaining treatment. Studies have consistently shown that physicians do not always follow ethical and legal guidelines when implementing withdrawals of life-sustaining treatment.[17] Nevertheless, the slippage is not believed to be serious enough to prohibit the refusal of life-sustaining treatment.

While it is still too early to draw definitive conclusions from the Oregon data, we know so far that despite fears that there would be a high rate of assisted suicide as a result of the law, it apparently is infrequently used, with fewer than 0.1 percent of deaths in Oregon taking place by assisted suicide.[18] Also, the right to a legalized form of suicide in Oregon does not seem to have encouraged suicide among young people in the state.[19]

Physicians who have reported assisting a suicide in Oregon appear to be complying with the requirements of the law,[20] and decisions to die by assisted suicide are apparently not being driven by poor education, lack of insurance, or inadequate palliative care.[21]

Still, as critics of assisted suicide have observed, there may be abuses not revealed by the Oregon data. We do not know whether patients in Oregon undergo an adequate psychiatric evaluation,[22] whether physicians know their patients well enough to judge the degree to which their decisions are voluntary,[23] or how careful Oregon physicians are in adhering to the law's requirement that the patient be terminally ill to qualify for assisted suicide. We also do not know whether abuses will become more common over time. We need more data from Oregon to fill out the picture.

3. *Decisions about physician-assisted suicide will typically occur in the privacy of the patient-physician relationship, making abuses undetectable.* Typically, proposals to legalize assisted suicide include a requirement that

the suicide be assisted by a physician. Indeed, Oregon's right to assisted suicide is a right to *physician*-assisted suicide. The requirement of physician participation serves a few important purposes. First, it is thought to protect against abuse. Physicians, it is felt, will be better able than family members or friends to detect a treatable depression. In addition, while it is not always possible to detect coercion, physicians can intervene if there is reason to suspect that the suicide request is motivated by the coercion of family or friends. Second, physicians can provide what is often the least painful and quickest method of assisted suicide: death by ingestion of medications they prescribe. Third, it is important to have physicians confirm the patient's diagnosis and prognosis, to ensure that the patient truly is terminally (or irreversibly) ill.

Still, it is argued, the additional safeguards provided by physician participation may not be sufficient.[24] In this view, regulation of assisted suicide must rely too heavily on physician self-regulation. Patients, with their physicians, would be able to decide about and commit suicide without outside involvement. Moreover, the confidentiality of discussions between patients and physicians would prevent adequate oversight. In other words, discussions and decisions about assisted suicide are inherently private in nature and therefore ill suited to public regulation. Either sensitivity to patient privacy would make it impossible to examine whether a decision to die was reached properly, or the necessary regulations to ensure propriety would be so intrusive that they would too greatly undermine patient confidentiality.[25] When the United States Supreme Court recognized a right to use contraception, it was concerned in large part by the specter of "the police [searching] the sacred precincts of marital bedrooms for telltale signs of the use of contraceptives."[26] Concerns about patient privacy and physician self-regulation are not as important with treatment withdrawals, it is argued, because they take place in the hospital, where there is a good deal of oversight.

This, too, is an important argument. However, there are several responses to the concern. First, third parties are often privy to decisions about assisted suicide.[27] Timothy Quill's patient, "Diane," had discussed her plans with her husband and children; so, too, did Janet Adkins, as well as many others whose deaths were assisted by Jack Kevorkian. The patient's family can often protect the patient's interests.[28] If a physician coerces a patient to agree to assisted suicide, family members may question the patient's sudden change of heart. Second, many treatment withdrawals and withholdings take place outside of a hospital, either in a nursing home, where oversight is poor, or at the patient's home. In these settings, the privacy of the patient-physician and other relationships can hide improper behavior. Nevertheless, we seem to be confident that physicians are not abusing their authority. If we can trust physician self-regulation with these treatment withdrawals, why can't we trust it with assisted suicide? Third, physicians who bend or ignore the law are subject to legal penalty. If a patient dies, and there is reason to suspect an unjustified act of euthanasia or assisted suicide, an autopsy can establish how the patient died. The physician will then need to be able to show that the suicide occurred in accordance with the law. The physician could create fraudulent entries in the patient's medical record, but frauds are difficult to conceal, especially since other evidence is likely to be inconsistent with the altered records. Finally, if the concern about the privacy of the patient-physician relationship rests on the fact that public evidence of a patient's consent does not reflect the subtle coercion that can occur in the privacy of patient-physician communications, that concern also applies just as much to decisions regarding the withdrawal or withholding of life-sustaining treatment.

4. *Demand for assisted suicide is predicated on concerns that are inherently subjective, making it difficult to develop sufficiently rigorous legal standards.* Many commentators argue that a right to assisted suicide cannot be limited in any meaningful way.[29] If assisted suicide is justified for the relief of suffering, individuals must decide whether they are appropriate candidates for assisted suicide, for only the individuals themselves can know whether their suffering has become intolerable. Accordingly, if assisted suicide were legalized, physicians or other potential assisters would have no basis for turning down a request for assisted suicide by any competent adult.

This is an important argument, but there is also an important response. Even if one accepts the view that individual autonomy should be the guiding principle for a right to assisted suicide, it does not follow that every competent adult should be allowed to choose assisted suicide.

Rather, Bayesian analysis[30] suggests that there should be some limits as to when assisted suicide should be available.[31] The response from Bayesian analysis works as follows. Assuming that a competent adult can choose assisted suicide, we still need to decide whether a person requesting suicide is truly competent. However, our methods for ascertaining competency are imprecise. Moreover, the imprecision of competency assessments has a greater impact when the likelihood of rational suicide is low. Consequently, when we try to decide whether a particular person requesting suicide is competent, we are likely to falsely conclude that the person is competent when the overall chances of irrational suicide are high. Thus, for example, if we believe that requests for suicide by patients who are not terminally ill are rarely going to be competent requests, we are highly likely to be wrong when we conclude that a person who is not terminally ill has competently chosen suicide. We are better off assuming that requests for suicide are incompetently made when they are made by persons who are not terminally ill.

Consider the following analogy: If a young, otherwise healthy adult refuses antibiotics for a bacterial pneumonia and offers no plausible reason for the refusal, we are likely to assume that the person is making an incompetent refusal of treatment. Even if the person seems competent, we are likely to conclude otherwise because it is difficult to imagine why a competent person would refuse treatment in such a situation.[32] In short, even if a theory for assisted suicide is based entirely on self-determination, objective limits on the circumstances under which a person can choose assisted suicide can still be justified.

5. *Is it possible to prohibit assisted suicide?* Heretofore, we have presented regulatory arguments against legalizing assisted suicide. Under those arguments, even if assisted suicide can be morally acceptable in principle, it cannot be implemented in a moral way in practice. There is also an important regulatory argument in favor of legalization. With this argument, the view is that even if assisted suicide is morally problematic, it cannot be effectively prohibited in practice, and the costs of prohibition outweigh the costs of legalization.

This argument is made for many morally controversial practices—regulation is chosen as an alternative to prohibition because the practices will occur in the face of prohibition, and the costs of a "black market" are viewed as too great. For example, this country's experiment with a prohibition on the manufacture, importation, or sale of alcoholic beverages lasted fourteen years until the public concluded that it was better to have alcohol available legally than illegally. Similarly, restrictions on gambling have loosened considerably in recent years, with many states joining Nevada in permitting lotteries, casinos, and other games of chance. With legalization, more people engage in the practice. On the other hand, the role of criminal or other undesirable elements is reduced. Thus, legalizing abortions results in more abortions, but it also nearly eliminates deaths of women from septic abortion.

With assisted suicide, studies have consistently shown that some physicians assist patients' suicides despite the illegality of their action.[33] In a significant number of these cases, it appears that physicians are not acting in accordance with the kinds of regulations that would be adopted if assisted suicide were permitted.[34] Proponents of assisted suicide argue that with legalization we can be more confident that assisted suicide will be employed appropriately. In other words, patients turn to the Jack Kevorkians of the world, and other physicians fail to follow safeguards like consulting with colleagues only when assisted suicide is illegal. Opponents of assisted suicide respond that legalization will result in more assisted suicides overall and that this would be worse than having a smaller number of suicides occur illicitly.

There is no obvious answer to this argument. Where one comes out depends on how problematic one views assisted suicide and on how problematic one views the costs of assisted suicide being performed illegally.

How to Proceed

Given the indeterminacy of the arguments on the question whether assisted suicide can be regulated, it is not clear how one should proceed. One could decide not to propose guidelines for assisted suicide on the ground that offering proposals would be seen as encouragement for laws permitting assisted suicide. One could decide instead to propose guidelines on the ground that assisted suicide is already occurring secretly and that it is better if physicians and/or other assisters have some guidance when they help individuals with suicide furtively.[35]

There is, however, an important development that argues in favor of model guidelines. Voters in Oregon have twice rejected arguments against legalizing assisted suicide, by progressively larger margins. The practice has begun to occur in the state. Although Oregonians are not receptive to a ban on assisted suicide, they may be receptive to modifications of their regulations for assisted suicide. In addition, if other states follow Oregon's lead and permit assisted suicide, model guidelines can help ensure that their laws are well drafted. The question then becomes, What regulations would be appropriate?

As a preliminary matter, an important question is whether assisted suicide should be legalized under limited circumstances, as in Oregon, or whether a state's legal prohibition should be maintained, with the creation of an affirmative legal defense to prosecution if assisted suicide is performed under limited circumstances.[36] (With an affirmative defense, a criminal defendant can justify excusal from conviction. For example, self-defense is an affirmative defense to a murder charge.) With legalization, physicians would be protected from prosecution as long as they acted in accordance with the statutory provisions. With an affirmative defense, physicians are more susceptible to prosecution, and they would bear the burden of persuading a jury that they met the requirements of the defense. Accordingly, physicians would be much more reluctant to assist a suicide under an affirmative defense approach than with legalization.[37] In other words, legalization poses a greater risk of too many assisted suicides; with an affirmative defense, there is a greater risk of too much patient suffering. Arguably, as a first step, it makes more sense to start with an affirmative defense, on the ground that we should proceed cautiously on a matter with so much at stake. On the other hand, the chilling effect of prosecutions with an affirmative defense approach will probably be very high, so high that it might not have much of an effect on physicians' practices. Indeed, even in states that prohibit assisted suicide, physicians know that they will escape prosecution or conviction if they assist suicides in reasonable situations. As a practical matter, then, we already have an affirmative defense system, and we know that physicians prefer to operate secretively under such a system.

For regulations to prevent abuse, it may be wise to err on the side of fairly conservative guidelines. In doing so, it is recognized that strict procedures protect patients from abuse by sacrificing the needs of patients who would be appropriate candidates for assisted suicide under the law. A two-week waiting period, for example, makes it more likely that the patient's request will be a firm one, but it also means that the patient's suffering will be prolonged even further. Moreover, if regulations are too strict, patients may turn to assisters who will help them in violation of the regulations. Given the risks of assisted suicide and the uncertainty regarding its implementation in the United States, however, approaches should be cautious. If experience indicates that more lenient regulation is appropriate, the guidelines can be relaxed.

In addition to deciding the content of guidelines or regulations, an important question is who should establish them. Legislators could legalize assisted suicide but leave it to a government agency or commission to draft regulations, just as Congress relies on the Department of Health and Human Services to issue regulations on federal health care matters. Legislators could also leave it to a nongovernmental organization to draft guidelines, just as the government turns to the Joint Commission for the Accreditation of Healthcare Organizations to promulgate guidelines for hospitals. Or, in the case of physician-assisted suicide, legislators could leave it to the medical profession to develop guidelines in the same way that courts rely on the profession to set standards for non-negligent medical practice.

In the end, legalization would likely involve a mix of several different approaches. A legislature, as in Oregon, can give general guidance but cannot possibly write a statute that covers all contingencies. A government health care agency or commission could then flesh out the law with more specific regulations. The profession could then bring clinical expertise to the regulations to flesh them out further. For example, the Oregon Death with Dignity Act requires the involvement of a "consulting physician" to confirm that the patient is terminally ill and is making a competent, voluntary, and informed decision.[38] The statute defines a consulting physician as someone "who is qualified by specialty experience to make a professional diagnosis and prognosis regarding the patient's disease."[39] A government agency could in turn give clearer guidance on when a physician is "qualified by specialty experience to make a professional diagnosis and prognosis." For example, the agency might require board certification or board eligibility in oncology if the patient is dying of cancer. The medical profession then would decide when a physician is board certified or board eligible in oncology (as it already does). In some cases, different entities can work together, as in Oregon, where a task force representing twenty-five health professional organizations, state agencies, and health systems published *Oregon's Death with Dignity Act: A Guidebook for Health Care Providers.*

Conclusion

There are serious questions about the regulatability of a legal right to assisted suicide. However, physician-assisted suicide has been legalized in Oregon. The question therefore is not so much whether assisted suicide, but how. Accordingly, it is important that rigorous safeguards be developed to ensure that the risks of abuse are minimized and to ensure that the experience with those regulations be monitored and assessed.

REFERENCES

1. See F. G. Miller, J. J. Fins, and L. Snyder, "Assisted Suicide and Refusal of Treatment: Valid Distinction or Distinction without a Difference" (Chapter 2); and K. Faber-Langendoen and J. H. T. Karlawish, "Ought Assisted Suicide Be Only *Physician* Assisted?" (Chapter 4).
2. In the *Martin* case, the Michigan Supreme Court rejected a wife's request to withdraw life-sustaining treatment from her severely brain-damaged husband because he had made specific statements about treatment in the event of permanent unconsciousness but not in the event of minimal consciousness. In re *Martin*, 538 N.W.2d 399 (Mich. 1991).
3. Y. Kamisar, "The 'Right to Die': On Drawing (and Erasing) Lines," *Duquesne Law Review* 35 (1996): 481; and T. J. Marzen, "'Out, Out Brief Candle': Constitutionally Prescribed Suicide for the Terminally Ill," *Hastings Constitutional Law Quarterly* 21 (1994): 799.
4. J. Lynn et al., "Defining the 'Terminally Ill': Insights from SUPPORT," *Duquesne Law Review* 35 (1996): 311; and E. Fox et al., "Evaluation of Prognostic Criteria for Determining Hospice Eligibility in Patients with Advanced Lung, Heart, or Liver Disease," *Journal of the American Medical Association* 282 (1999): 1638–1645.
5. Kamisar, "The 'Right to Die.'"
6. Commission on the Acceptability of Termination of Life of the Royal

Dutch Medical Association, "Seriously Demented Patients" (1993), in J. Griffiths, A. Bood, and H. Weyers, *Euthanasia and Law in the Netherlands* (Amsterdam: Amsterdam University Press, 1998), 134–139.

7. Given these considerations, a number of proposals would allow assisted suicide for any patient who is incurably ill and suffering greatly, whether or not the patient is terminally ill. In addition, some proposals would allow both assisted suicide and euthanasia.

8. A. Meisel, *The Right to Die*, 2d ed. (New York: John Wiley and Sons, 1995), §§ 8.10, 8.13, 9.39.

9. W. J. Curran et al., *Health Care Law and Ethics*, 5th ed. (New York: Aspen Law and Business, 1998), 628–630.

10. D. Orentlicher, "The Legalization of Physician-Assisted Suicide: A Very Modest Revolution," *Boston College Law Review* 38 (1997): 443; and D. Orentlicher, "The Legalization of Physician-Assisted Suicide," *New England Journal of Medicine* 335 (1996): 663–667. Similarly, the granting of the right to vote at age eighteen does not reflect any real moral difference between eighteen-year-olds and seventeen-year-olds. Rather, the distinction between adults and minors does a *generally* good job of sorting individuals with the maturity and judgment to cast a ballot from individuals who lack that maturity and judgment.

11. Orentlicher, "The Legalization of Physician-Assisted Suicide."

12. Y. Conwell and E. D. Caine, "Rational Suicide and the Right to Die: Reality and Myth," *New England Journal of Medicine* 325 (1991): 1100, 1101.

13. C. Gomez, *Regulating Death: Euthanasia and the Case of the Netherlands* (New York: Free Press, 1991), 135–139; and H. Hendin, *Seduced by Death: Doctors, Patients, and the Dutch Cure* (New York: W. W. Norton, 1997).

14. In about half of the cases without an explicit and contemporaneous request, the patient had in a previous phase of his or her illness expressed a wish for euthanasia should suffering become unbearable, or the decision had been discussed with the patient but the patient's wishes had not been expressed explicitly and persistently. In the other half of cases, the patients had not expressed prior wishes and were incompetent but were very close to death and clearly suffering greatly. P. J. van der Maas et al., "Euthanasia and Other Medical Decisions Concerning the End of Life," *Lancet* 338 (1991): 669, 672; and P. J. van der Maas et al., "Euthanasia, Physician-Assisted Suicide, and Other Medical Practices Involving the End of Life in the Netherlands, 1990–1995," *New England Journal of Medicine* 335 (1996): 1669, 1701. With the incompetent patients, it is quite possible that euthanasia was performed against what would have been their wishes. Whether this violates the spirit of the Netherlands guidelines is unclear. If one rests the right to euthanasia solely on considerations of patient autonomy, then there is a violation of the spirit of the guidelines. If, on the other hand, one rests the right to euthanasia also on considerations of the patient's current best interests, then some might argue that there need not be a violation of the spirit of the guidelines.

15. R. A. Epstein, *Mortal Peril: Our Inalienable Right to Health Care?* (Reading, Mass.: Addison-Wesley, 1997), 321–322.

16. As indicated in Hendin, *Seduced by Death*, the Dutch studies indicate that cases in violation of the safeguards involve patients for whom (1) there was good evidence that euthanasia was desired or (2) evidence of the patient's wishes was unavailable, the patient was incompetent and near death, and euthanasia was provided to relieve great suffering.

17. See D. Orentlicher, "The Limits of Legislation," *Maryland Law Review* 53 (1994): 1255, 1280–1301; and SUPPORT Principal Investigators, "A Controlled Trial to Improve Care for Seriously Ill Hospitalized Patients: The Study to Understand Prognoses and Preferences for Outcomes and Risks of Treatments (SUPPORT)," *Journal of the American Medical Association* 274 (1995): 1591.

18. A.D. Sullivan, K. Hedberg, and D. W. Fleming, "Legalized Physician-Assisted Suicide in Oregon—The Second Year," *New England Journal of Medicine* 342 (2000): 598–600 (reporting that 0.06 percent of deaths in Oregon in 1998 and 0.09 percent in 1999 occurred by physician-assisted suicide).

19. B. Coombs Lee and J. L. Werth Jr., "Observations on the First Year of Oregon's Death with Dignity Act," *Psychology, Public Policy, and Law* 6 (2000): 268–290.

20. Ibid.; and Sullivan et al., "Legalized Physician-Assisted Suicide in Oregon."

21. Sullivan et al., "Legalized Physician-Assisted Suicide in Oregon," 602.

22. Coombs Lee and Werth, "Observations on the First Year of Oregon's Death with Dignity Act"; and H. Hendin, K. Foley, and M. White, "Physician-Assisted Suicide: Reflections on Oregon's First Case," *Issues in Law and Medicine* 14 (1998): 243, 251–254.

23. W. J. Smith, "Dependency or Death? Oregonians Make a Chilling Choice," *Wall Street Journal*, 25 February 1999.

24. D. Callahan and M. White, "The Legalization of Physician-Assisted Suicide: Creating a Regulatory Potemkin Village," *University of Richmond Law Review* 30 (1996): 1.

25. Ibid.

26. *Griswold v. Connecticut*, 381 U.S. 479, 485 (1965).

27. F. G. Miller, H. Brody, and T. E. Quill, "Can Physician-Assisted Suicide Be Regulated Effectively?" *Journal of Law, Medicine, and Ethics* 24 (1996): 225.

28. To be sure, family members do not always have the patient's best interests at heart.

29. Y. Kamisar, "Physician-Assisted Suicide: The Problems Presented by the Compelling Heartwrenching Case," *Journal of Criminal Law and Criminology* 88 (1998):1121.

30. Bayesian analysis takes into account the fact that diagnostic tests and other medical assessments are not always accurate. B. J. McNeil, E. Keller, and S. J. Adelstein, "Primer on Certain Elements of Medical Decision Making," *New England Journal of Medicine* 293 (1975): 211–215. A person may have heart disease even with a normal EKG (a falsely negative EKG), and another person may not have heart disease even with an abnormal EKG (a falsely positive EKG). All medical tests have false negative and false positive results. What this means is that if one tests positive for cancer, one's chances of cancer are higher than before the test, but still not 100 percent. Similarly, if one tests negative for cancer, one's chances of cancer are lower than before the test, but still not zero. To determine a patient's actual risk of cancer after a cancer test, physicians need to know two things: the accuracy of the test (how often the test is falsely positive or falsely negative) and the likelihood that the patient had cancer before the test was performed (the prior probability of cancer or the prevalence of cancer in people like the patient). For example, if a patient had a 10 percent chance of cancer before being tested, and the test is accurate 90 percent of the time (90 percent sensitivity and specificity), then a test that is positive for

cancer indicates that the patient now has a 50 percent chance of cancer. If the patient had a 60 percent chance of cancer before being tested, then a positive test means that the patient now has a 93 percent chance of cancer. And if the patient had a 1 percent chance of cancer before being tested, a positive test would mean that the patient now has an 8 percent chance of cancer. Just as tests for heart disease or cancer are inaccurate some of the time, so are psychiatric assessments of a patient's competence to make medical decisions. Thus, if 10 percent of patients who desire suicide are making a competent choice of suicide, and psychiatric assessments of competence are accurate 90 percent of the time, a conclusion that a patient is competent means that the patient still only has a 50 percent chance of making a competent choice of suicide.

31. Epstein, *Mortal Peril.*
32. A. R. Jonsen, M. Siegler, and W. J. Winslade, *Clinical Ethics: A Practical Approach to Ethical Decisions in Clinical Medicine,* 3d ed. (New York: McGraw Hill, 1992), 15, 47, 62.
33. D. E. Meier et al., "A National Survey of Physician-Assisted Suicide and Euthanasia in the United States," *New England Journal of Medicine* 338 (1998): 1193; and A. L. Back et al., "Physician-Assisted Suicide and Euthanasia in Washington State," *Journal of the American Medical Association* 275 (1996): 919.
34. E. J. Emanuel et al., "The Practice of Euthanasia and Physician-Assisted Suicide in the United States: Adherence to Proposed Safeguards and Effects on Physicians," *Journal of the American Medical Association* 280 (1998): 507.
35. S. Heilig et al., "Physician-Hastened Death: Advisory Guidelines for the San Francisco Bay Area from the Bay Area Network of Ethics Committees," *Western Journal of Medicine* 166 (1997): 370.
36. J. A. Tulsky, A. Alpers, and B. Lo, "A Middle Ground on Physician-Assisted Suicide," *Cambridge Quarterly of Healthcare Ethics* 5 (1996): 33.
37. Miller et al., "Can Physician-Assisted Suicide Be Regulated Effectively?"
38. *Oregon Death with Dignity Act,* § 3.02.
39. Ibid., § 1.01(3).

Six

TIMOTHY E. QUILL, M.D., BARBARA COOMBS LEE, P.A., F.N.P., J.D., AND SALLY J. NUNN, R.N.

Palliative Treatments of Last Resort: Choosing the Least Harmful Alternative

CLINICIANS, ETHICISTS, POLICY MAKERS, and lawyers generally agree that comprehensive palliative care is the standard of care for the dying[1] and that any intervention that is likely to hasten death should only be considered as a last resort when life has become intolerable to the patient in the face of unrestrained efforts to relieve suffering.[2] There is also general agreement that patients should receive sufficient treatment of their pain,[3] even in doses that risk hastening death, and that patients have the right to forgo life-sustaining treatment even if their desire is for a quick and certain death.[4] More recently, terminal sedation and voluntarily stopping eating and drinking have been proposed as alternatives to physician-assisted suicide for those whose suffering cannot be addressed by standard pain management and the stopping of life supports.[5] Although these practices are more clinically and ethically complex than is generally recognized,[6] they can be offered without violating current laws and are felt by some to be morally superior to physician-assisted suicide as options of last resort.

This chapter uses the descriptive phrase "prescribing a potentially lethal medication" to classify what many would categorize as physician-assisted suicide. Any act where death is intentionally sought by the patient might meet the technical definition of suicide.[7] But the meaning of suicide connotes an act of self-destructiveness, which is why those in medicine work so hard to prevent it. Therefore, for the purposes of this paper we use descriptive terminology to categorize all of these last-resort acts. Since any of these acts could result in a hastened death, their moral and clinical evaluation should always take into consideration the clinical context, the proportionate degree of suffering, the absence of less harmful alternatives, and the nature of the decision-making process.

When a patient expresses a wish to die, this should begin an exploration of the adequacy of palliative care, including assessments of pain management, depression, anxiety, family burnout, and spiritual and existential issues.[8] For patients who are genuinely ready to die, for whom suffering is intolerable despite comprehensive palliative efforts, an exploration of methods for easing death can begin. The methods will be determined by the patient's clinical situation; the values of the physician, patient, and family; and the status of current law. Table 6.1 outlines current methods that may hasten death. Standard pain management, including accelerating doses of opioids when needed to relieve terminal crescendos of pain or shortness of breath, and forgoing life-sustaining treatment have gained widespread legal and ethical acceptance.[9] Terminal sedation and voluntarily stopping eating and drinking are more ethically complex but also probably legal.[10] Prescribing potentially lethal medications remains ethically controversial and is generally illegal, although no clinician has ever been successfully prosecuted for participating with beneficent intent.[11] The first four options can be practiced openly, with good documentation and consultation, whereas the latter must be carried out in secret, except in Oregon, which regulates this practice.[12] Clinicians faced with these difficult decisions should be aware of all of these options, including their indications, risks, benefits, and likely outcomes, and how to discuss them with patients and families.

In this chapter we present relatively straightforward clinical cases to illustrate situations when each of the interventions might be chosen. Each clinical scenario is followed by a brief commentary about some of the clinical issues raised. References are provided for those who want more information about the legal, ethical, and policy implications. The predictable availability of some of these options can be valuable to patients who have witnessed a bad death and fear a similar experience. Most will not request such assistance if they receive state-of-the-art palliative care, but some want to know potential options. Knowledge of the range of possibilities can also help clinicians better respond to the rare patients whose pain and suffering becomes intolerable, without violating their own values, and without abandoning patients to continue unacceptable suffering or to violent attempts to end life. Clinicians who care for severely ill patients must become aware of these options and decide which ones they are willing to provide as a last

Table 6.1   Palliative Interventions of Last Resort:

Options Currently Under Consideration in Order of Increasing Legal and Ethical Uncertainty

Intervention	Certainty of Death	Patient Competence	Physician Involvement	Legal Status	Ethical Consensus
Standard pain management	Uncertain and unintended by either patient or physician	Not required	Yes	Legal	Yes
Forgoing life-sustaining therapy	+ Dialysis +/- Vent, feeding tube, steroids, insulin	Not required	Usually	Legal	Yes
Voluntarily stopping eating and drinking	Certain (requires time and discipline)	Required	Desirable, but not necessary	Legal	Growing consensus
Terminal sedation: heavy sedation to escape pain, shortness of breath, other severe symptoms	Certain if fluids withheld, which is standard practice	Not required	Yes	Legal	Growing consensus
Prescribing a potentially lethal medication (with knowledge of patient intent)	Uncertain (patient may not take at all, or not take as directed; medication may not work)	Required	Yes–prescribing No–administering	Generally illegal, but unlikely to result in prosecution	No, but widespread public support
Voluntary active euthanasia	Certain	Required	Yes	Illegal, and likely to be prosecuted	No

resort. Since all of these choices are less than ideal, the challenge is to find the least harmful alternative given the patient's circumstances and the values of the patient, family, and clinicians involved.

Clinical Examples of Potential Last-Resort Intervention

STANDARD PAIN MANAGEMENT

A sixty-eight-year old man who has metastatic small-cell lung cancer is having excruciating pain and is near death. He initially responded to a combination of radiation and chemotherapy, achieving a three-year remission during which he was able to continue to work and live his usual life. His disease recurred four months previously, and he elected a palliative approach after consultation with his primary care doctor and his oncologist. His extensive, painful bony metastases have been his main symptomatic challenge, and his pain has been well controlled with a combination of high-dose, around-the-clock oral opioids, palliative radiation, and nerve blocks. He has prepared for death by having long talks with his family and clergy and feels that he has no remaining "unfinished business." He now weighs eighty pounds and is largely bedbound. His pain has begun to accelerate and is now usually rated as eight on a ten-point scale. He does not want to die but is willing to accept the risk of sedation and earlier death that might come from increasing doses of pain medicine. After consultation with the hospice medical director and a specialist in pain management, the primary care physician agrees to increase both his around-the-clock and hourly as-needed opioid doses by 25 percent per day until the patient says that his pain is adequately controlled or, if the patient cannot report pain, he appears comfortable.

The first day produced no demonstrable effect on his pain or sedation, but on the second day the patient was very sleepy, but arousable, and appeared relatively free of pain. The physician continued the same amount of opioid treatment but shifted the mode of administration from oral to transcutaneous because the patient was unable to reliably swallow. The patient died two days later. He appeared comfortable for his last forty-eight hours, although he was largely unresponsive.

Commentary: This activity meets the criteria for standard pain management and has wide acceptance within medical ethics, palliative medicine, religion, and the law.[13] Giving adequate analgesia to patients who are dying has wide social acceptance. For most of the patient's illness, his pain was well controlled, and he was fully alert and functioning despite the use of high-dose opioids. When his pain accelerated toward the end of his life, both patient and physician were willing to take the risk of death as an unintended side effect, but it was not a hidden or explicit purpose. The patient's suffering was proportionately severe enough to warrant taking the risk of unintentionally accelerating death. Although good pain management can usually be achieved without sedation and without shortening life, sometimes the pain is so severe or the patient is so frail that the risk of accelerating death is real. When the patient lapsed into a sedated state, the dose of opioid was neither increased nor decreased, and the side effect of sedation was accepted as proportionately necessary to control his pain.

WITHDRAWAL OF LIFE SUPPORTS

A fifty-six-year old man developed a malignant brain tumor three years previously. He initially responded to a combination of surgery, radiation, and chemotherapy. Although his cognitive abilities were diminished such that he could no longer do his work as an accountant, he had found joy in spending time with his great passion of painting. In fact, his altered brain unleashed additional creativity and innovation in his painting, which he saw as a small compensating blessing for his many losses. Over the last six months, his tumor had begun to grow rapidly, and he began to have terrifying seizures where his thoughts would be jumbled, and he would feel paranoid and attacked. During his seizure-free times, he began talking in earnest about being ready to die. He was treated with a variety of antiseizure and antidepressant medications, as well as dexamethasone to minimize brain swelling. Unfortunately, there was little relief. Once he tried to end his suffering by jumping into Lake Ontario in the middle of winter and was saved at the last second. This led to twenty-four-hour supervision to prevent such "suicidal" actions.

During one of his many hospitalizations, his physician realized that dexamethasone was probably prolonging his life, and the patient could choose to discontinue it. After discussion with his neurologist, psychiatrist, family, and an ethicist, it was decided that it was both morally acceptable and clinically appropriate to raise the question with the patient, who was informed of the possible choice and the likely outcome (his wished-for death). Any pain that emerged in the process could be managed aggressively in line with standard pain management. Once informed of this possibility, the patient immediately refused further dexamethasone. He did not want a waiting period—from his perspective, he had waited too long already. Within twelve hours of stopping the dexamethasone, he went into a deep coma (probably from a combination of brain swelling and iatrogenic adrenal insufficiency). Fortunately, he had no pain or agitation. He died peacefully twenty-four hours later with his family in attendance.

Commentary: The patient's right to refuse treatment, including treatments that may be life sustaining, such as ventilators, dialysis, feeding tubes, insulin, or dexamethasone, has wide legal and ethical acceptance.[14] This right holds even if the patient wishes to die and could live indefinitely with the treatment, provided that the patient is fully informed about the alternatives, and has mental capacity to understand the decision. Families can generally make these decisions on behalf of a patient who has lost mental capacity, provided there is a clear consensus that such an act reflects the patient's values, previously stated wishes, and best interests.[15] Because such decisions frequently result in the patient's death, clinicians should be forthright about evaluating such requests, carefully assessing the patient's mental capacity, information about all palliative care alternatives, and the proportionate presence of suffering. All three of these domains should be fully explored before a life-sustaining therapy is discontinued. This particular patient's wish to die was initially considered an irrational sign of psychopathology, until it was realized that he was within his rights to stop life supports. This opened up a very serious, open-minded conversation among patient, family, physicians, and the health care team that had previously been impossible.

VOLUNTARILY STOPPING EATING AND DRINKING
An eighty-three-year-old woman was admitted to a nursing facility one year after experiencing a major cerebrovascular accident which left her with a dense hemiparesis, although she retained cognition. Her husband died ten years earlier, but she had family living in town, including two sons, a daughter, and many grandchildren, who helped support her and brought her great joy. With a combination of home health care and family support, she was able to stay at home for the first year after her stroke. Unfortunately, her skilled nursing needs eventually became more than could be managed at home, and she was admitted to a skilled nursing facility. Her other chronic medical problems included degenerative joint disease, osteoporosis, and stable coronary artery disease.

Six months after the admission, after extensive discussions with her family, her doctor, and clergy, she stopped all of her medicines other than pain relievers and adopted a palliative approach. Her goal was to achieve a quicker end to what had become for her an interminable dying process. Her care at the nursing facility was supplemented by a hospice team. She initially felt elated by the decision and began the process of saying goodbye by telling all of her life stories to her children in tape-recorded interviews. She would accept only those treatments devoted to her immediate comfort—no antibiotics, no disease-related treatments, no hospitalization, no tests of any kind. After three months of rich and meaningful preparation, all of the stories had been told, and she had stabilized off all medicines.

She then began talking in earnest about wanting to die and trying to find a way to achieve this end without jeopardizing her family or her physician. Being a lifelong Unitarian, she had no personal moral objection to voluntarily hastening death, but she refused to compromise anyone in her family or her physician, given the current state of the law. She read a newspaper account of David Eddy's mother's choice of stopping eating and drinking[16] and immediately began exploring it with her family and physician. There was an initial worry by several family members and staff that it would be a long, painful process of starvation and dehydration, but her doctor researched the literature and found some data about cancer patients dying this way, which she found reassuring.[17] Several members of the nursing home staff were unable to accept her choice and were reassigned to other patients.

After multiple meetings among the patient, family, clergy, hospice staff, and the nursing home team, she began the process. Her family visited every day in rotating shifts, and each was able to say goodbye in his or her own way. The patient was initially very talkative and had a special word for each of her children and grandchildren. On about day six, she became more sleepy and intermittently confused. There was some uncertainty about whether to stop the process because she could no longer consent, or whether she was suffering enough in her confusion to be sedated, but the physician, family, and staff felt that their obligation was to continue the course chosen by the patient and to hold off on sedation. The nursing staff kept her mouth moist and her skin well creamed. Her favorite music played constantly in the background. The staff was prepared to provide sedation if she became agitated or clearly uncomfortable, but this proved unnecessary. She was in a coma for the final three days of the fifteen-day process, and she died quietly in her family's presence.

Commentary: Voluntarily stopping eating and drinking usually leads to death within one to three weeks.[18] Since the physician's role is clearly indirect (ensuring an informed decision and awareness of palliative care alternatives, and then addressing uncomfortable symptoms), this process does not require a change in the law. Since stopping eating and drinking is viewed as a variant of stopping life-sustaining treatment, it is theoretically available to those, such as the patient described, who are not imminently terminal. The process requires substantial self-discipline and cooperation from family and health care providers. The substantial delay between initiation and death may be prohibitive for some patients with severe, immediate symptoms. There may also be substantial palliative care challenges as the process unfolds. Many patients, who fear that the health care system will not respect their decision to choose death no matter how severe their suffering, find this possibility reassuring because it theoretically does not require "permission" from or participation by health care providers. In fact, especially if the patient is in a health care institution, the team must agree at a minimum not to interfere with the process. Ideally, clinicians participate in the initial decision and then commit to palliate symptoms throughout the course.

TERMINAL SEDATION

A thirty-five-year old man had acquired immunodeficiency syndrome (AIDS) for more than ten years. He had been near death several times over the last five years and had been in an AIDS hospice at the time protease inhibitors became available. The addition of protease inhibitors gave him a new lease on life for more than two years, emerging from recurrent infections and severe wasting to feeling robust, gaining weight, and returning to his work as a designer. However, over the last nine months his disease again began progressing in spite of numerous medication adjustments. He started losing weight again, developed AIDS-related enteropathy, and began to lose his sight as a result of his long-standing CMV retinitis. This time, despite numerous changes in his anti-retroviral regimen, there was no reprieve. He was again admitted to a residential hospice. He accepted that he was dying and was more fearful of suffering severely than of death itself. His physician promised to remain responsive no matter what happened. The patient was very fearful of AIDS dementia and wanted to be reassured that he could be sedated if he became severely confused or agitated.

His initial time in the hospice program was comfortable and meaningful, as he had healing contact with family, friends, and clergy. As death approached, he developed high fevers, rigors, and increasing shortness of breath. These symptoms were treated with a morphine infusion and acetaminophen, but there was no medical workup or antibiotic treatment. As the dose of morphine was increased to try to relieve his symptoms, he became delirious and agitated. The dose was decreased, and he awoke but was very uncomfortable. The patient requested that the doctor help him escape from his agony. The doctor offered to sedate him to unconsciousness and then withhold further treatments including intravenous fluids. The patient was reassured that the dose would be increased until he appeared to be resting comfortably and that it would not be discontinued or cut back until he died. The doctor and patient discussed the decision with close family and friends, as well as the caregivers in the hospice program. A consensus was reached that this was the best of the available options. It would allow the patient to achieve a wished-for death without violating the law or forcing him to suffer unnecessarily. He was put on a midazolam infusion, which was titrated upward until he achieved a sedated state and then maintained at that level. He died within twenty-four hours.

Commentary: Terminal sedation has been proposed as an alternative to physician-assisted suicide for severely symptomatic, terminally ill patients that does not require changes in the law.[19] The patient is sedated to unconsciousness to relieve severe physical suffering and then allowed to die of dehydration or some other intervening complication. Terminal sedation is theoretically considered to be a combination of aggressive symptom management (sedatives to treat unbearable symptoms) and withdrawal of life-sustaining therapy (fluids, nutrition, and other treatments). When considered as an aggregate act, terminal sedation is morally complex for those who believe in an absolute prohibition to intentionally hastening death.[20] The practice differs technically from euthanasia in that the dose of medication is maintained but not increased once sedation is achieved, and there is no subsequent intervention to accelerate death such as the introduction of a muscle-paralyzing agent.

Terminal sedation allows health care providers to respond to a much wider range of suffering than would physician-assisted suicide even if legalized, since the latter would be restricted to competent terminally ill patients who are capable of self-administration. Terminal sedation has been used to respond to troubling syndromes such as terminal delirium, where patients lose mental capacity at the end. The facts that terminal sedation is not immediately lethal and requires a team to administer are felt by some to be important safeguards.[21] Guidelines for the practice have been proposed, but relatively little is known about the range and extent of the actual practice.

PRESCRIBING A POTENTIALLY LETHAL MEDICATION

A fifty-nine-year-old man was diagnosed with oropharyngeal cancer two years previously. The tumor was too large to be resected, so he was treated with a combination of chemotherapy and radiation. He responded well to the treatment, and after recovering from the side effects of radiation on his esophagus, he had a relatively asymptomatic year during which he was able to work at his usual job. His tumor recurred inside his mouth and in his neck, making it hard to swallow his secretions. He wanted to live as long as his symptoms could be adequately managed and then to die as quickly and painlessly as possible. He was particularly afraid of suffocation, which he had seen in a coworker who died of emphysema. A feeding tube was inserted with the knowledge that it could be stopped at a time of his choosing, and he would then be allowed to die. His pain was well controlled with around-the-clock administration of sustained-release morphine. He was admitted to a home hospice program, and his children moved in to be primary caregivers.

His time on hospice was very meaningful, with regular visits from members of his church congregation, friends, hospice nurses, aides, and volunteers. As he became weaker, he considered stopping the feeding tube but chose not to because he still found reason to keep living in his family contact. His tumor began to grow around his carotid artery and eventually eroded into it, resulting in profuse bleeding both inside his mouth and outside his neck. He was terrified of suffocation and of bleeding to death in front of his family. He asked for enough medication to "put me out of my misery." He agreed to stop his feeding tube but felt that the wait for him to dehydrate to death would be too long given his current acutely deteriorating condition. He was offered terminal sedation so that he could escape his suffering but remained fearful of bleeding out and suffocating and not being able to tell his caregivers about his subjective state. He was also worried about the impact on the family of watching him bleed to death. His family understood and accepted his decision and was willing to support him in the process if the physician would provide a prescription for barbiturates. After discussing the situation with his practice partners, the physician reluctantly but knowingly provided him with a lethal amount of barbiturates in a prescription ostensibly intended for insomnia. That evening the patient took the entire amount with his family present, went into a deep sleep, and died quietly.

Commentary: This doctor and patient chose prescription of potentially lethal medication because the other last-resort options could not satisfactorily address his particular situation.[22] After a long period of excellent palliation, this patient became acutely symptomatic as death approached. Although he was on life-sustaining treatment, stopping eating and drinking (in his case, artificial feeding) was not quick-acting enough to be responsive to his particular clinical circumstances. Terminal sedation was also possible, but he feared suffocation while sedated and feared being unable to alert his caregivers of his distress. He was also concerned about the impact on his family were he to bleed to death while sedated. The physician, after having private conversation about the clinical situation with his colleagues, reluctantly provided a prescription for barbiturates that could hasten death if taken all at once. Because of legal fears, the physician was not physically present to respond to complications but was available to the family by telephone should problems arise. Maintaining the patient in a terminally sedated state was the physician's backup plan, but the patient died without complications.

Discussion

Although the case studies presented here portray clear distinctions among the five specific palliative interventions, in practice both the clinical indications and the practices may blur. Categorization may depend on specific circumstances and may be subject to interpretation. For example, the distinction between terminal sedation and voluntary active euthanasia is based in part on whether the sedative is maintained or increased once sedation is achieved, and whether a lethal injection is given. It is also often based on the physician's intent to hasten death, which is subjective, often ambiguous, and never absolutely knowable.[23] Reasonable observers might differ in their categorization of terminal sedation in terms of intent.[24] Similarly, what begins as voluntarily stopping eating and drinking in an alert, capable patient may become withholding life supports from an incompetent patient as obtundation occurs. If the patient subsequently becomes delirious in this terminal phase, this practice might have to be followed by terminal sedation. Experienced clinicians could easily think of numerous other complex examples where the health care team and the family might be extremely challenged to find an adequate approach.

Each of these interventions alone or in combination may have a small place at the very end of life in the care of severely ill patients for whom palliative care is failing. Only in the standard pain management case was death clearly unintended by both patient and physician—the risk of death was understood, given the grave symptomatic condition of the patient, but it was not the goal of either party. With the other four interventions, death was the inevitable outcome, and was actually being sought by the patients. Although the physician's purpose in participating in these alternatives is to respond to human suffering, the decision-making process should include acknowledgment that death is inevitable. In any and all of these interventions, the physician must ensure the adequacy of palliative care, a full exploration of alternatives, the patient's mental capacity, and the proportionate presence of suffering.

Standard pain management and stopping life-sustaining therapy are standards of care, and all clinicians should be willing to provide them. Even though voluntarily stopping eating and drinking and terminal sedation are legal, they should be considered more extra-ordinary options, considered only when no acceptable alternatives are available and when both patient and physician consider participation to be moral. Providing potentially lethal medication remains illegal in most states. It should be exceedingly rare, given only on request from the terminally ill patient whose suffering is intolerable, when other alternatives are inadequate to address the patient's clinical circumstances or are incompatible with fundamental patient values. When physicians unilaterally choose not to participate in any of the latter three options, they have an obligation to search for acceptable alternatives with the patient. Ethics and palliative care consultations may be helpful in the search for common ground. If a mutually acceptable approach cannot be found, the patient and family should be given the option of transferring care to another physician.

REFERENCES

1. Council on Scientific Affairs of the American Medical Association, "Good Care of the Dying Patient," *Journal of the American Medical Association* 275 (1996): 474–478; American Board of Internal Medicine End of Life Patient Care Project Committee, *Caring for the Dying: Identification and Promotion of Physician Competency.* (Philadelphia: ABIM, 1996); ABIM End-of-Life Patient Care Project Committee, "Caring for the Dying: Identification and Promotion of Physician Competence," Educational Resource Document (Philadelphia: ABIM. 1996); American Medical Association Council on Ethical and Judicial Affairs, "Decisions Near the End of Life," *Journal of the American Medical Association* 276 (1992): 2229–2233; Council on Scientific Affairs, American Medical Association, "Good Care for the Dying Patient," *Journal of the American Medical Association* 275 (1996); 474–478; M. J. Field and C. K. Cassel, eds., *Approaching Death: Improving Care at the End of Life* (Washington: National Academy Press, 1997); K. M. Foley, "Pain, Physician-Assisted Suicide, and Euthanasia," *Pain Forum* 4 (1995): 163–178; and T. E. Quill, *Death and Dignity: Making Choices and Taking Charge* (New York: W. W. Norton and Co., 1993), 1–255.
2. T. E. Quill, B. Lo, and D. Brock, "Palliative Options of Last Resort: A Comparison of Voluntarily Stopping Eating and Drinking, Terminal Sedation, Physician-Assisted Suicide, and Voluntary Active Euthanasia," *Journal of the American Medical Association* 278 (1997): 2099–2104.
3. See Note 1.
4. L. Gantz, "Withholding and Withdrawing Treatment: The Role of the Criminal Law," *Law, Medicine, and Health Care* 15 (1988); 231–241; A. Meisel, "Legal Myths about Terminating Life Support," *Archives of Internal Medicine* 151 (1991): 1497–1502; D. K. Miller, "Achieving Consensus on Withdrawing or Withholding Care for Critically Ill Patients," *Journal of General Internal Medicine* 7 (1992): 475–480; H. Brody et al., "Withdrawing Intensive Life-Sustaining Treatment—Recommendations for Compassionate Clinical Management," *New England Journal of Medicine* 336 (1997): 652–657; R. F. Weir and L. Gostin, "Decisions to Abate Life-Sustaining Treatment for Nonautonomous Patients: Ethical Standards and Legal Liability for Physicians after Cruzan," *Journal of the American Medical Association* 264 (1990): 1846–1853; and W. C. Wilson et al., "Ordering and Administration of Sedatives and Analgesics during the Withholding and

Withdrawal of Life Support from Critically Ill Patients," *Journal of the American Medical Association* 267 (1992): 949–953.

5. Quill et al., "Palliative Options of Last Resort"; R. D. Troug et al., "Barbiturates in the Care of the Terminally Ill," *New England Journal of Medicine* 327 (1991): 1678–1681; N. I. Cherney and R. K. Portenoy, "Sedation in the Management of Refractory Symptoms: Guidelines for Evaluation and Treatment," *Journal of Palliative Care* 10 (1994): 31–38; V. Ventifridda et al., "Symptom Prevalence and Control during Cancer Patients' Last Days of Life," *Journal of Palliative Care* 6 (1990): 7–11; J. L. Bernat, B. Gert, and R. P. Mogielnicki, "Patient Refusal of Hydration and Nutrition: An Alternative to Physician-Assisted Suicide or Voluntary Active Euthanasia," *Archives of Internal Medicine* 153 (1993): 2723–2727; L. A. Printz, "Terminal Dehydration, a Compassionate Treatment," *Archives of Internal Medicine* 152 (1992): 697–700; and F. G. Miller and D. E. Meier, "Voluntary Death: A Comparison of Terminal Dehydration and Physician-Assisted Suicide," *Annals of Internal Medicine* 128 (1998): 559–562.

6. Quill et al., "Palliative Options of Last Resort"; T. E. Quill, "The Ambiguity of Clinical Intentions," *New England Journal of Medicine* 329 (1993): 1039–1040; and T. E. Quill, R. Dresser, and D. W. Brock, "The Rule of Double Effect: A Critique of Its Role in End-of-Life Decision Making," *New England Journal of Medicine* 337 (1997): 1768–1771.

7. T. L. Beauchamp, "Suicide," in *Encyclopedia of Bioethics*, vol. 2, ed. W. T. Reich (New York: Simon and Schuster, 1995), chap. 3; and *Oxford English Dictionary* (New York: Oxford University Press, 1971), 912.

8. T. E. Quill, "Doctor, I Want to Die. Will You Help Me?" *Journal of the American Medical Association* 270 (1993): 870–873; S. D. Block and J. A. Billings, "Patient Requests to Hasten Death: Evaluation and Management in Terminal Care," *Archives of Internal Medicine* 154 (1994): 2039–2047; F. Ackerman, "The Significance of a Wish," *Hastings Center Report* (July-August 1991): 27–29; and M. A. Rie, "The Limits of a Wish," *Hastings Center Report* (July-August 1991): 24–27.

9. See Notes 1 and 4.

10. See Note 5.

11. Quill, *Death and Dignity*; *Vacco v. Quill*, 117 S.Ct. 2293 (1997); *Washington v. Glucksberg*, 117 S.Ct. 2258 (1997); R. A. Burt, "The Supreme Court Speaks—Not Assisted Suicide, but a Constitutional Right to Palliative Care," *New England Journal of Medicine* 337 (1997): 1234–1236; and A. Alpers and B. Lo, "Physician-Assisted Suicide in Oregon: A Bold Experiment," *Journal of the American Medical Association* 274 (1995): 483–487.

12. Alpers and Lo, "Physician-Assisted Suicide in Oregon."

13. Quill et al., "The Rule of Double Effect;" and see Note 1.

14. See Note 4.

15. Weir and Gostin, "Decisions to Abate Life-Sustaining Treatment for Nonautonomous Patients."

16. D. M. Eddy, "A Conversation with My Mother," *Journal of the American Medical Association* 272 (1994): 179–181.

17. R. M. McCann, W. J. Hall, and A. Groth-Juncker, "Comfort Care for Terminally Ill Patients," *Journal of the American Medical Association* 272 (1994): 1263–1266.

18. Quill et al., "Palliative Options of Last Resort"; Bernat et al., "Patient Refusal of Hydration and Nutrition"; Printz, "Terminal Dehydration, a Compassionate Treatment"; and Miller and Meier, "Voluntary Death."

19. Quill et al., "Palliative Options of Last Resort"; Troug et al., "Barbiturates in the Care of the Terminally Ill"; Cherney and Portenoy, "Sedation in the Management of Refractory Symptoms"; and Ventifridda et al., "Symptom Prevalence and Control during Cancer Patients' Last Days of Life."

20. Quill et al., "Palliative Options of Last Resort"; Quill et al., "The Rule of Double Effect"; and J. A. Billings and S. D. Block, "Slow Euthanasia," *Journal of Palliative Care* 12 (1996): 21–30.

21. Cherney and Portenoy, "Sedation in the Management of Refractory Symptoms."

22. Quill, *Death and Dignity*; and Quill et al., "Palliative Options of Last Resort."

23. Quill, "The Ambiguity of Clinical Intentions"; and Quill et al., "The Rule of Double Effect."

24. Quill et al., "Palliative Options of Last Resort"; and Billings and Block, "Slow Euthanasia."

Seven

JAMES A. TULSKY, M.D., RALPH CIAMPA, S.T.M., AND ELLIOTT J. ROSEN, ED.D.

Responding to Legal Requests for Physician-Assisted Suicide

IN 1998 FIFTEEN TERMINALLY ILL Oregon residents ended their lives with overdoses of medications supplied legally by their physicians.[1] Eight others received prescriptions they never used. These numbers likely represent the tip of the iceberg of patients who consider physician-assisted suicide at some point in their illness, only some of whom will ask their physicians directly for help.

Several thoughtful pieces have been written to guide physicians who receive requests for physician-assisted suicide.[2] All address the major medical, psychosocial, and spiritual issues confronting dying patients who consider ending their own lives. Emanuel describes a protocol that prohibits physicians from ever assisting in dying. Block and Quill, although more sympathetic to physician-assisted suicide, wrote at a time when assisted suicide was illegal in all states.

The Oregon referendum legalizing physician-assisted suicide dramatically alters this landscape. Physicians are faced with new ethical challenges as they weigh requests from patients. For example, even when legal, requests for physician-assisted suicide will continue to surface as vague expressions of the wish to die rather than as direct inquiries. Does legalization allow or perhaps even compel physicians to raise the possibility of assisted suicide as a treatment option? This chapter will examine how the physician's response to requests for assisted suicide may change in an era of legalization, articulate some of the resulting conceptual challenges, describe the domains of suffering that motivate patients to request physician-assisted suicide, and provide practical advice to physicians facing such requests.

What Changes When Assisted Suicide Becomes Legal?

Legalization of assisted suicide may change the nature of communication between physicians and patients regarding decisions at the end of life. Discussion of physician-assisted suicide is no longer taboo and becomes, in fact, one of the many options to be freely considered. Furthermore, when assisted suicide is legal, dissatisfied patients are empowered to bring their requests to other physicians, who may not know the patient as well. Six of the patients described in the recent Oregon experience approached one or two physicians prior to finding someone willing to fulfill their request.[3]

Some patients will view physician-assisted suicide as a right that the physician merely facilitates and thus change the doctor-patient interaction from a therapeutic encounter to one of negotiation. That is, physician-assisted suicide may become a service that some patients may expect on demand. Even if such patients appear uninterested in hearing about other options, physicians must be able to respond empathetically to a patient's concerns and try to understand and address the issues that are leading that person to this decision. Physicians in Oregon appear to recognize this fact and, since the introduction of physician-assisted suicide, have heightened their skills in palliative care.[4]

Some Conceptual Issues

With little experience to guide us, some may view informed consent as the likely model for discussions about assisted suicide.[5] In this model, the physician discusses the risks, benefits, likely outcomes (e.g., not always death, as in the case of a botched suicide), and alternatives. In fact, such a model may apply to a discussion of options to end one's life, after extensive counseling and palliative care have been provided. However, in many cases, requests for physician-assisted suicide appear to be almost the converse of classic informed consent. The patient sets the agenda and asks the physician to consent to the request. If the physician disagrees, the conflict is likely to be over values rather than simply information. Furthermore, the extreme emotional nature of the topic challenges rational decision making.

Because of these complexities, we recommend that these discussions be viewed in a more collaborative or therapeutic model of communication. This model focuses on the biopsychosocial concerns of the patient and, through empathic listening and emotional support, helps the patient identify a solution that addresses these concerns. When considering some of the troubling questions that arise, we may begin with informed consent but must recognize the limitations of that model, as we have learned with regard to advance directives and the forgoing of life-sustaining medical treatments.[6]

ASSESSING DECISION-MAKING CAPACITY

There is general agreement that patients requesting physician-assisted suicide must have decision-making capacity. However, we have traditionally viewed a desire to end one's own life as a possible sign of depression or some other pathological mental state. Typically, we endeavor to protect patients from harming themselves. Yet depression in the dying patient may be qualitatively different.

On the one hand, identifying depression in the terminally ill may be deceptively simple.[7] On the other hand, the presumption that clinically depressed patients are wholly incapable of making rational requests to end their lives seems far too facile and may simply avoid dealing with the complexities of suffering. Terminally ill patients that meet criteria for clinical depression may nevertheless be making a rational decision to die. Moreover, since antidepressant medication may take weeks to be effective, such a trial of medication for someone suffering intolerably and desiring death, whose life expectancy is a matter of days, may not be a realistic option. Nevertheless, these issues are extremely complex. Some requests, even in end-stage patients, are motivated by treatable depressions, and therapies such as amphetamines may clear depression rapidly. Clarifying these issues often warrants expert consultation.[8]

DISCLOSURE OF THE OPTION

Physicians are ethically obligated to explore, in a meaningful way, a patient's request for physician-assisted suicide. If such a request is sustained despite the physician's attempts at presenting other viable choices, the doctor should discuss the patient's options under the law. However, discussing physician-assisted suicide with a patient who does not request this option explicitly is problematic.

Under the strictest definition of informed consent, physicians would appear to be obligated to disclose to all terminally ill patients the option of physician-assisted suicide. At the very least, requirements for truth telling would incline one to disclose the options that are available to the terminally ill patient who is looking for a way out of intractable suffering. For example, many terminally ill patients may not be aware that they have other choices such as terminal sedation or the voluntary stopping of eating and drinking—legal and, for many, an ethically acceptable means to hasten death. The withholding of such information does not allow a patient to make a fully informed decision and would violate a reasonable formulation of the notion of informed consent.

However, does describing these alternatives connote endorsement, and is there any risk that by raising the issue a patient may become motivated to commit an action that would not have occurred otherwise? Clearly, simply mentioning options does not imply endorsement of these options. In medicine, we routinely describe to patients options that we consider unwise, but we do so in the interest of full disclosure. In an environment in which assisted suicide is legal, is asking about suicide suggestive or coercive?

In the course of caring for dying patients, physicians frequently explore issues of depression and suicidality. To not do so with the patient who is thinking seriously about this option would be to leave the patient alone with his or her thoughts and therefore vulnerable to increased anguish. Furthermore, asking a patient who one suspects is thinking about suicide to talk about these feelings is more akin to reflecting or naming the patient's feelings than to encouraging suicide. For example, we do not worry that a physician's statement to a patient, "You seem depressed," will induce depression where none existed. Rather, the doctor is clarifying an interpretation of the patient's mood. Perhaps a better analogy is to informing patients that they may stop a life-sustaining medical treatment. Many people find the knowledge that they could end their suffering to be liberating, thus actually giving them the strength to go on.

GIVING A RECOMMENDATION

Traditionally, information giving in the informed-consent process is thought to be value-neutral. In reality, however, information can be framed in many different ways that will have different implications for decision making.[9] Furthermore, some argue that neutrality is not beneficial in the informed-consent model, that physicians aid informed consent by providing an opinion.[10] However, when doing so, physicians must also be clear that patients understand the recommendation to be an opinion and not a statement of medical fact. Full informed consent typically includes a recommendation by the health care professional. In addition to acquiring information on risks and benefits, most patients want to know what their doctor thinks is best for them. While they may choose to reject this opinion, it is one more piece of data upon which to base a decision.

Physician-assisted suicide, however, seems to be different. Should

physicians ever disclose their personal views on physician-assisted suicide, particularly to patients with life-threatening illness? It may be in
the patient's interest to know early that a physician is in favor of or
categorically opposed to the practice so that the patient has the opportunity to consider changing doctors. On the other hand, a physician's
focus on his or her own beliefs may shift the attention away from the
patient. For example, telling patients, too early in the conversation,
that one is opposed to assisted suicide on principle may deter them
from disclosing their deepest concerns.[11]

In addition, we must be mindful of the power of medical authority
when talking to patients. Patients fear their doctors' disapproval and
may not easily distinguish the fine line between open and appropriate
disagreement and coercion. Patients may construe a physician's abrupt
declaration of opposition to physician-assisted suicide as a conversation
stopper and form of abandonment.[12] Many patients are searching simply for someone to talk to or to help ease their dying.

Avoiding a sense of abandonment is one of the central dilemmas
facing physicians who receive requests for physician-assisted suicide.
Physicians who are personally opposed to assisted death and cannot
comply with a patient's request do not want their patients to feel that
they are not "with them" through the end. Such physicians must find
a way to demonstrate that commitment even when they will not assist
with the patient's death. Since suicide is the final act of a patient's life,
not being there "at the end" may carry considerable symbolic meaning.
Of course, simply writing a prescription is no assurance that a patient
will not feel, or be, abandoned. But physicians must be attentive to the
nuances of abandonment experienced by patients in this situation and
must seek effective ways to reassure the patient of supportive care.

We have considered so far whether physicians must disclose the option of assisted suicide or should share their views in opposition to the
practice. But can a physician ever recommend assisted suicide to a patient? Can a doctor ever tell a patient that in light of his unmitigated
suffering, taking his own life would be the best choice? As stated earlier,
physicians are expected to educate patients about their options and to
aid them in decision making by offering a recommendation that is
medically sound and appears to be compatible with the patient's values
and goals for care. Recommendations help put decisions into a framework of physicians' experiences and their best guess as to how the disease and treatments will play out.

However, a recommendation to commit suicide, even if legal, seems
inappropriate. Even if one believes that it is in the physician's role to
assist with suicide, it seems a significant step beyond that role to recommend a hastened death. Given the general prohibition against kill-

ing, there seems to be a difference between hesitatingly helping a patient end his or her life and encouraging a patient to die. Furthermore, no matter how many patients they care for, physicians can claim no more authority about the personal experience of death and suffering than can patients.

When trying to decide how much to disclose to a patient about options for physician-assisted suicide, the risks of unintended coercion and abandonment must be viewed in tension with risks of violations of obligations to tell the truth. Certainly, routine terminal care is not likely to include descriptions of all options. Furthermore, no physician, even when practicing in a jurisdiction that allows physician-assisted suicide, should ever encourage a patient to hasten death. The physician should describe, where it is legal, the process by which assisted suicide is handled and help the patient understand what the act would involve in medical and social terms. Nevertheless, when confronted with a patient who wants to die, the physician is also obliged to let the patient know that while physician-assisted suicide is a legal option, other options exist as well, such as terminal sedation and/or voluntary stopping of eating and drinking. Physicians who are willing to assist in suicide ought to make it clear that they will help the patient, if necessary, but that their job is to try to help the patient find a way to make that option unnecessary.

THE ROLE OF GOOD COMMUNICATION

Good communication in response to a patient's request can have a tremendous impact not only on the choices the patient will make, but also on the quality of dying. A conversation about a patient's desire to end his or her life can be a form of therapy, so discussion itself may be palliative. It is an opportunity to address the patient's greatest fears and concerns and respond to these issues. The converse is also true: poor communication can be damaging.

A physician's communication skills and the willingness to enter into such a vital conversation are key elements in nonabandonment; thus, it would be wise for professionals to explore their own beliefs before engaging patients in conversation. While patients and families are likely to be sensitive to a physician's ambivalence about providing assisting in dying, a doctor's own clarity about the issue will enhance this important therapeutic encounter.[13] Described below are the factors that bring patients to express a wish for an early death and potential physician responses to these expressions of suffering. In constructing appropriate responses, we wish to emphasize that listening and empathetically exploring, without necessarily resolving issues, are by far the most important skills.

Domains of Suffering

The deepest suffering motivates suicide. Generally, pain, fatigue, or dyspnea alone are insufficient reasons for an individual to desire to end his or her own life, given the potential for their palliation.[14] Several key domains of suffering, described below, appear to torture patients enough to lead them to request physician-assisted suicide and are deserving areas of exploration by physicians who encounter such patients. This chapter focuses on the role of physicians because they are the only professionals empowered by law to fulfill requests for physician-assisted suicide. Furthermore, they frequently are the first to learn of patients' concerns in the context of a request for physician-assisted suicide. However, many physicians are ill prepared to address these domains and must enlist their colleagues in chaplaincy, nursing, social work, psychology, and other fields, to respond appropriately.

"I'M A BURDEN."
This statement reflects concerns about dependency. Is the perceived burden financial, physical, or emotional? The provider must listen empathetically, explore the concern, and attempt to mitigate the burdensome aspects of care when possible. Family members may be engaged to reassure the patient that caring is not a burden. In fact, patients may see that committing suicide may actually create an additional burden.[15]

On the other hand, patients' perceptions of burden are frequently real and cannot be resolved through additional resources. Even when loving families are willing to provide the care, some patients may not want to see them spending their time and resources in this manner. For example, they may not want their legacy to include the interruption of a child or grandchild's education because that person needed to stay home and care for them.

If burden is created by an inflexible system that does not provide adequate financial support or appropriate medical care, does that change the legitimacy of the request for that patient? Requests for physician-assisted suicide by impoverished patients with limited access to care are particularly problematic. Physicians may have a moral obligation to help families in such situations identify and demand the necessary resources.

"NO ONE CARES ABOUT ME."
Such troubled assertions usually reflect feelings of depression, isolation, or abandonment. These can be the most profound sentiments leading to a desire for death. Oftentimes, such feelings originate from family difficulties in handling the patient and the illness. Engagement

of the family and other appropriate health care professionals, such as a social worker or a member of the clergy, is vital at this juncture.

"I CAN NO LONGER TOLERATE THE PAIN."

Many patients suffer intolerable physical pain, and clinicians have an ethical obligation to explore whether all palliative options have been exhausted.[16] In those rare cases when symptoms such as pain, dyspnea, or nausea cannot be controlled, the physician may wish to discuss terminal sedation. Terminal sedation, of course, is not without its difficulties, among them questions of competency, creation of a slippery slope, and the belief by some that the process is merely "slow euthanasia."[17]

"I FEEL LIKE I'M GOING CRAZY."

Dying patients may experience frightening and disorienting psychiatric symptoms such as depression and delirium. These may be a reaction to the emotional stress of the experience, the underlying disease, or treatment. Addressing such symptoms is beyond the scope of this chapter, and an effective response may require the input of psychiatric or palliative care consultants. It is also important to take responsibility for listening carefully to what patients are saying, even if meaning is not obvious or is conveyed in seemingly strange ways.[18]

"NONE OF THIS IS EVER GOING TO GET BETTER."

This expression of hopelessness, although a defining symptom of depression, may also be an expression of reality. The belief—and the likelihood—that nothing will change raises the question of how much suffering patients must endure. Simple acknowledgment and quiet, accepting support of the patient's inevitable and appropriate grief may be most helpful at this point. While patients must be afforded the hope of palliative care and pain control, other options within the patient's control, such as voluntarily ceasing eating and drinking or terminal sedation, should also be raised. Knowing about such options may give patients comfort even if they never employ them.

"LIFE HAS LOST MEANING FOR ME."

Clinicians struggle with this statement because its subjectivity appears to pose an insurmountable problem. Life-threatening illness may trigger deep spiritual crises for patients, who wonder why this illness has befallen them or feel abandoned by God. Patients may also have overwhelming feelings of remorse that life has been worthless or, in some cases, feel satisfied that they have completed their life's work and now have nothing more for which to live. The clinician's role is to explore, empathize, express support, and refer to an appropriate counselor. Such profound questions about life's purpose are often best handled by a clergy member, who can provide a spiritual framework within which the patient can find some meaning to face death less fearfully. Similarly, patients who seriously consider physician-assisted suicide often wonder about the acceptability of such a choice in their religious tradition and what repercussions such an act might have on their spiritual well-being. Patients with these concerns should also be encouraged to consult clergy. Some patients will request that physicians join them in prayer or other spiritual ceremonies.

"I'M TIRED OF DYING."

Some patients, after completing the preparatory work of dying and saying their good-byes, will see no reason to continue for weeks or months in their current state, even without overwhelming symptoms. Clinicians may try to confront a failure of imagination on the patient's part and identify continued goals for living. However, physicians may also need to question their own imagination when they cannot accept a patient's readiness to die. If the patient were receiving life-sustaining treatment, such as dialysis, we may more readily accept a decision to withdraw treatment. In such situations, the possibility of an escape through physician-assisted suicide may actually provide the strength to keep going. According to published data about the first year of the Oregon law, more than one-third of the patients who went through the lengthy process never used their prescription for a lethal overdose.[19]

Practical Suggestions for Engaging in the Dialogue

1. IDENTIFY, ACKNOWLEDGE, AND CLARIFY THE REQUEST.

Physicians should allow patients an opportunity to fully share their thoughts and feelings. When one seems reasonably certain that a patient is asking for physician-assisted suicide, it is appropriate to address the request directly. A physician might respond, "I understand that you are saying there are circumstances under which you might want to end your life or hasten your death. How were you hoping I might be able to help you?"

In other cases, patients may vaguely suggest a request, to which physicians might respond, "You have referred several times recently to 'wishing it were all over' and 'wondering if you can hold on any longer.' Though you haven't quite said it, it sounds like you are thinking that there are alternatives to waiting for death to come naturally. I would be interested in knowing what is on your mind in that regard."

Finally, in some cases, the physician will want to explore what appear to be suicidal thoughts that have not been communicated directly but might be implied. For example, "You have shown great courage in living with the burdens of your illness. I want to support you in that struggle in every possible way. I am also wondering if you ever think about a point at which the pain and struggle would be more than you want to continue bearing, and whether you have given any thought to what your alternatives might be. Those are also questions you can think about with me."

2. EXPLORE THE PATIENT'S CONCERNS AND ADDRESS PHYSICAL,
PSYCHOSOCIAL, AND SPIRITUAL SUFFERING.

It may help to classify the patient's concerns into one of the domains of suffering described earlier. One can begin such a discussion by asking, "What is the worst part of your condition right now for you?" If that does not lead to a clear vision of what makes the patient's suffering intolerable, one might tell the patient, "In my experience, other people's thoughts about ending their lives seem to be connected to one or more of a number of factors: their belief that their pain will never get under control, their feelings of despair about a burden they have put upon their loved ones, or a sense that they can find no meaning in continuing life. Do your thoughts fall into one of those categories?"

3. DEVELOP WITH THE PATIENT AN UNDERSTANDING OF THE GOALS OF
TREATMENT, FOCUSING NOT ONLY ON PHYSICAL SYMPTOMS BUT ALSO
ON CAPACITY TO LIVE MEANINGFULLY AS DEFINED BY THE PATIENT.

A physician can discuss with the patient what can reasonably be expected of treatment and develop the goals of that treatment collaboratively. This may include managing physical symptoms to facilitate other goals. For example, patients often report that there is still a special event, such as the birth of a child or a wedding, that itself would define a continuing desire to live. If such a patient is suffering uncontrolled physical symptoms which prompt the wish to die, managing those physical symptoms in anticipation of the important event becomes a fundamental treatment goal. One can say to the patient, "I know how important it is for you to get to the wedding. I'm not sure how well we can manage these symptoms until then, but why don't we try? Afterward, we can certainly reconsider what we're going to do next."

4. IMPLEMENT THE TREATMENT PLAN AND MONITOR THE PATIENT'S
COURSE FOR POINTS AT WHICH INTERVENTIONS NO LONGER SEEM
COMPATIBLE WITH THOSE GOALS. IF GOALS CANNOT BE ACHIEVED,
SEARCH FOR LESS HARMFUL ALTERNATIVES.

If initial efforts are not successful in relieving suffering, a physician may consult experts in palliative care and other appropriate professionals.

However, if a patient has requested physician-assisted suicide contingent on the success of the agreed-upon treatment goals, and the interventions are failing to achieve those goals, the physician must plot a new course. It is necessary to begin a dialogue with the patient that acknowledges that the goals of treatment cannot be achieved and that all options for palliative care have been exhausted. At this point it is useful to search for less harmful and more universally acceptable options. For example, if pain is the problem, one can promise to increase the analgesics until relief or escape. If the patient is on life-sustaining treatments, these can be discontinued. One also can consider whether terminal sedation or stopping eating and drinking are possibilities for the doctor and patient.

5. IF INTEREST IN SUICIDE REMAINS, ACKNOWLEDGE AND CLARIFY THE REQUEST, BE EXPLICIT ABOUT THE LEVEL OF PARTICIPATION WHICH IS CONSCIENTIOUSLY ACCEPTABLE, AND EXPRESS THIS TO THE PATIENT.
A few patients will continue to request physician-assisted suicide despite the best efforts of the primary physician and expert consultants. The physician should clarify exactly what the patient is requesting. Does the patient want a prescription, or is the patient envisioning more active involvement on the part of the physician? In many ways, this may be the most difficult point in the process. When the patient believes that all other options available have been exhausted, the physician must address directly the hard question of what he or she is willing to do in order to assist a patient to end life.

Some physicians, of course, will be willing to participate in physician-assisted suicide under appropriate circumstances. They might say to the patient, "In our state the law allows me to prescribe medications which you could use to end your life. I believe there might be circumstances under which doing so would be a part of my professional commitment to relieve suffering. So I would be open to considering that option further with you."

Others will be unwilling to prescribe lethal medication but may feel comfortable raising terminal sedation or voluntary stopping eating and drinking as other options: "Although our state laws do allow doctors to prescribe medication which might be used to end your life, it is against my personal conscience to participate in that way. If we can think of no other way to relieve your suffering, perhaps we should discuss ways in which your own actions, short of taking a lethal medication, might hasten your death and bring your suffering to an end. For example, if you were to completely stop eating and drinking, your body would succumb to a natural death within two to three weeks. People who choose this option experience little discomfort and maintain their dignity and control."

Others will acknowledge the legal option but express unwillingness to ever participate, including offering terminal sedation or advising on stopping eating and drinking. Such physicians might state that "although the law allows physicians to prescribe medication that could be used to end your life, my own conscience does not allow me to do that. But you could no doubt find other physicians in our community who would consider that possibility with you and perhaps give you that option under carefully considered circumstances." Physicians who are comfortable doing so ought to refer the patient to a physician who might be more willing to participate.

When physicians are unwilling to assist in a patient's request, they must be exceedingly careful to avoid any sense of abandonment. "Although I cannot in good conscience prescribe a lethal medication as the law allows, I want to assure you that I will not abandon you in your approaching death. I will continue to think with you about your many legitimate concerns and to help find persons to respond to those concerns. And if a point should come where relief of your physical pain or distress requires medicines that could also hasten your death, then I would be willing to go on relieving your pain, if I clearly knew that is what you want."

6. OFFER ALL RELEVANT INFORMATION ABOUT
LEGAL FRAMEWORK AND REALISTIC OPTIONS.

At this point, the informed consent model applies most directly. Patients must understand their options under the law. This includes knowing how to go about assisted suicide under applicable statutes (e.g., waiting periods, witnesses, effective medications, and dosages) as well as other options such as terminal sedation and voluntary stopping of eating and drinking. It also includes addressing tough issues such as what to do if the attempted suicide fails or if patients change their mind midstream. If at all possible, such discussions should be held with the patient and other family members, since the latter are likely to be directly involved in either the act of assisting in the dying or expected to have some role in whatever subsequently ensues.

7. CLARIFY YOUR OWN STANCE ON THE PATIENT'S
REQUEST AND SPEAK WITH COLLEAGUES.

Physicians should not go it alone. Many of the emotions felt by the patient, such as hopelessness and frustration with current therapies, are shared by the doctor. When patients express a wish to die, physicians may also feel abandoned.

We have attempted to consider how physicians might respond to patients' requests to end their lives. Legalization of physician-assisted suicide places worrisome new demands on physicians. The willingness to explore one's own response to suffering, finitude, death, and hope is crucial to any profound participation in these conversations. If legal physician-assisted suicide becomes more common, firsthand reports from others may provide more sophisticated direction to physicians facing a changing moral frontier. But what such legislation will certainly do is forge a new covenant between caregiver and patient.

REFERENCES

1. A. E. Chin et al., "Legalized Physician-Assisted Suicide in Oregon: The First Year's Experience," *New England Journal of Medicine* 340 (1999): 577–583;

2. S. D. Block and J. A. Billings, "Patient Requests to Hasten Death: Evaluation and Management in Terminal Care," *Archives of Internal Medicine* 154 (1994): 2039–2047; L. L. Emanuel, "Facing Requests for Physician-Assisted Suicide: Toward a Practical and Principled Clinical Skill Set," *Journal of the American Medical Association* 280 (1998): 643–647; and T. E. Quill, "Doctor, I Want to Die. Will You Help Me?" *Journal of the American Medical Association* 270 (1993): 870–873.

3. Chin et al., "Legalized Physician-Assisted Suicide in Oregon."

4. M. A. Lee and S. W. Tolle, "Oregon's Assisted Suicide Vote: The Silver Lining," *Annals of Internal Medicine* 124 (1996): 267–269; and S. Tolle, "Care of the Dying: Clinical and Financial Lessons from the Oregon Experience," *Annals of Internal Medicine* 128 (1998): 567–568.

5. Emanuel, "Facing Requests for Physician-Assisted Suicide."

6. P. M. Dunn and W. Levinson, "Discussing Futility with Patients and Families," *Journal of General Internal Medicine* 11 (1996): 689–693; J. M. Teno and J. Lynn, "Putting Advance-Care Planning into Action," *Journal of Clinical Ethics* 7 (1996): 205–214 and J. A. Tulsky et al., "Opening the Black Box: How Do Physicians Communicate about Advance Directives?" *Annals of Internal Medicine* 129 (1998): 441–449.

7. H. M. Chochinov et al., "'Are You Depressed?' Screening for Depression in the Terminally Ill," *American Journal of Psychiatry* 154 (1997): 674–676.

8. Block and Billings, "Patient Requests to Hasten Death."

9. A. Tversky and D. Kahneman, "The Framing of Decisions and the Psychology of Choice," *Science* 211 (1981): 453–458.

10. A. Caplan, "Neutrality Is Not Morality: The Ethics of Genetic Counseling," in *Prescribing Our Future*, ed. D. Bartels, B. LeRoy, and A. Caplan (New York: Aldine de Gruyter, 1993), 149–165; and T. E. Quill and H. Brody, "Physician Recommendations and Patient Autonomy: Finding a Balance between Physician Power and Patient Choice," *Annals of Internal Medicine* 125 (1996): 763–769.

11. P. Maguire et al., "Helping Cancer Patients Disclose Their Concerns," *European Journal of Cancer* 32A (1996): 78–81.

12. T. E. Quill and C. K. Cassel, "Nonabandonment: A Central Obligation for Physicians," *Annals of Internal Medicine* 122 (1995): 368–374.

13. M. J. Edwards and S. W. Tolle, "Disconnecting a Ventilator at the Request of a Patient Who Knows He Will Then Die: The Doctor's Anguish," *Annals of Internal Medicine* 117 (1992): 254–256.

14. Chin et al., "Legalized Physician-Assisted Suicide in Oregon."

15. E. J. Rosen, "Commentary: A Case of 'Terminal Sedation' in the Family," *Journal of Pain Symptom Management* 16 (1998): 406–407.
16. American College of Physicians, "Position Paper: Ethics Manual, 4th edition," *Annals of Internal Medicine* 128 (1998): 576–594.
17. Rosen, "Commentary: A Case of 'Terminal Sedation' in the Family"; J. A. Billings and S. Block, "Slow Euthanasia," *Journal of Palliative Care* 12 (1996): 21–30; and G. P. Smith, "Terminal Sedation as Palliative Care: Revalidating a Right to a Good Death," *Cambridge Quarterly of Healthcare Ethics* 7 (1998): 382–387.
18. M. Callanan and P. Kelly, *Final Gifts: Understanding the Special Awareness, Needs, and Communication of the Dying* (New York: Poseidon Press, 1992).
19. Chin et al., "Legalized Physician-Assisted Suicide in Oregon."

Eight

FRANK DAVIDOFF, M.D.

Lessons from the Dying

Introduction

Our only son died in 1985 of metastatic bowel cancer. He was twenty-six. During his final illness the question of assisted suicide never came up, partly, I suppose, because he died before the issue had risen to the level of national consciousness it is at now, some fifteen years later, and partly because he died relatively quickly. Besides, his condition kept changing too unpredictably during the three months between diagnosis and death for us even to think about such a possibility. Toward the end, though, he was working so hard to deal with intractable symptoms—unremitting intestinal obstruction, uncontrollable ascites, unrelenting hiccoughs, violent waves of nausea, weakness, wasting—that it would have been entirely understandable and, perhaps, acceptable to us if he had asked to be helped to die sooner than he did. From that experience we learned a number of lessons about dying that bear directly on the question of assisted suicide. The principal lesson is that dying is extremely hard work.

Two years later the son of close friends committed suicide. He was twenty-one. From that experience we learned other lessons about dying that bear on assisted suicide. The principal lesson is how bitter the legacy of suicide can be.

It's hazardous, of course, to generalize from limited experience, particularly the deaths of young people. But when it comes to something

as profoundly complex as assisted suicide, the lessons learned from personal experience can contribute uniquely to our understanding of the
issues. For what it's worth, then, this essay considers what certain lessons from the dying teach us about assisted suicide.

Dying Is Hard Work

Dying is obviously not a great deal of work for someone who is shot in
the head or killed instantly in an auto accident. But I can assure you
that dying from a progressive major illness is extremely difficult. In fact,
I've rarely seen anyone work as hard—physically or emotionally—at
anything as our son did during his final days and weeks of dying. It is
impossible to appreciate how hard a dying person is working—fighting
symptoms, then accepting them; trying to understand what is happening; concentrating intensely on staying in control, then trying to let
go—unless and until you've sat by their bedside as we did, hour after
hour, day after day. Doctors, ethicists, and others almost *never* have that
experience with dying patients, which seriously limits their understanding about the work of dying; nurses, on the other hand, get to know a
lot about it.

I've also been struck by how much dying has in common with childbirth, which is not such a strange connection as might seem. The two
are, after all, mirror images: Childbirth ushers someone into the world,
dying ushers them out. What's more, childbirth, like serious illness,
carries a finite risk of dying; both involve intense pain; both require
hard emotional and physical work. Given the similarity, it's curious that
the language clearly recognizes the hard work of giving birth by calling
it "labor" but fails to capture the enormous effort involved in dying.
Instead we have terms like "failing," "losing strength," "giving up the
ghost"—the language of weakness, torpor, passivity—for the process
of dying. Medicine has long accepted the legitimacy of midwives and
obstetricians, specialists whose primary role is to help women through
the labor of childbirth. These experts aren't expected to cure most of
their patients of anything. Given the similarity between childbirth and
dying, and the enormous physical and emotional needs of dying patients, it also seems curious that a medical specialty, analogous to obstetrics, that focuses on care of the dying, and is not expected to cure
patients, has somehow never managed to emerge.

The Myth of the Easy Death

Sherwin Nuland's 1994 book, *How We Die*, is a recent, and rare, attempt
to take an honest look at the realities of dying. The blurb on the dust

jacket tells us that "there is a vast literature on death and dying, but there are few reliable accounts of the ways in which we die. . . . *How We Die* is not meant to prompt horror or terror but to demythologize the process of dying."[1]

Dying has, in fact, been seriously mythologized and for a very long time. Victorian novels supported the fantasy that death was easy, a matter of gently letting go; classically, the dying simply "turned their face to the wall." Although exceptions exist (the recent play *W;t* is a notable one), modern novels and films have generally perpetuated that myth with their sanitized versions of dying from illness: Patients are seen neatly tucked up in bed, saying their good-byes; the bleeding and the retching, the purulent sputum and the smells, the unrelenting pain and fatigue, the gasping for air of real dying are nowhere to be found; rarely are loss of control, assaults on dignity, or failure to reach closure dealt with in a convincing way.

How can it be that the realities of dying have managed to go unrecognized for so long? How can it be that a meaningful professional response to those realities has been so slow in coming? Denial is the obvious answer, and denial certainly is at the heart of the problem.[2] But denial is also reinforced at every turn by a system that allows doctors, and others, to tune out the process of dying. Medicine's role (with the partial exception of obstetrics) is held to be synonymous with cure or, in the case of chronic disease, management. Once the problem becomes "unmanageable," i.e., once death is inevitable, the system in effect allows, even encourages, doctors to disengage, to turn on their heels and walk away, to get back to their "real" work of curing the sick. The usual medical expression is, "I'm sorry; there's nothing more we can do." This view is, of course, extraordinarily ironic since it is at this point that the hard work of dying really begins, and the need for highly skilled help is greatest. But once the problem is "dying," the responsibility for care in our current system is immediately shifted from doctors to others: nurses, social workers, family members, and, ultimately, undertakers.

People involved in quality improvement are fond of saying that "a system is perfectly designed to get the results it gets." To the extent that's true, it is not an accident, then, that care of the dying in the United States (and elsewhere) is in bad shape: The current care system is perfectly designed to deliver inadequate care to dying patients. What are the operating principles that account for its inadequacy? First, scientific medicine is made possible only by stripping diseases of their personal meanings, which allows diseases to be modeled as abstract, generalizable concepts. It can hardly be surprising, therefore, if these

abstractions literally become more meaningful, more real, to scientifi-
cally trained physicians than the live patients they care for.[3]

Second, in contradistinction to the way physicians model disease as
neutral, abstract concepts, patients always assign metaphorical meaning to their illnesses.[4] Taking responsibility for helping people die a
"good" death inevitably means wading into a swamp of emotional, social, and moral meanings, not to mention powerful emotional issues.
Thus, physicians who engage fully in the care of dying patients can
anticipate the need to come to grips with their own sense of powerless-
ness, as well as anger, guilt, and shame in themselves and in patients
and their families. Why is this happening? Why wasn't more done? Why
was so much done? What will the family (or my colleagues) think?
Where were you when we needed you? Who's making decisions around
here? Whose life is it anyway?

Third, serious, often ambiguous, legal questions—negligence, abandonment, complicity, even murder—are always lurking in the background. Fourth, physicians are used to being in charge, in control, protected. Unfortunately, the usual professional protections don't apply
when it comes to care of the dying, which gives doctors additional incentives to opt out. Fifth, the current lack of training that would equip
doctors to take on this burden is also not an accident; it reflects the
same avoidance behavior among faculty, including the writers of medical textbooks,[5] as found among practicing clinicians. And finally, at
least until recently, no one has been willing to pay for palliative care.

The Spectrum of Care for the Dying

Few would disagree that medicine's basic purpose is to heal—to make
whole again. Medicine's purpose is also described as the relief of suffering. The two definitions are congruent if suffering is understood to
mean damage to patients' integrity, or the wholeness of their "personhood," as Eric Cassell has suggested.[6] The damage to personhood experienced by an otherwise healthy young patient with, say, pneumococ-
cal pneumonia is, of course, quite different from that of someone dying
of congestive heart failure, or AIDS, or cancer. But if medicine's purpose is to be the same for everyone, as it must, then doctors' obligation
to help preserve or restore personhood for a dying patient is at least
as great as the obligation to prescribe penicillin for a patient with pneumonia.

The problem, of course, is that there is no penicillin for dying. What
medicine can provide for someone who is dying of terminal illness depends on the patient, the illness—and the care system. Patients who

are dying have to work hard because they need to deal with so many problems all at once. Physical illness forces people in on themselves; the outside world drops away; pain, or lack of mobility, or inability to breathe, or fever, or physical ugliness becomes the center of their universe. Thinking, work, pleasures are eroded. And illness always takes on social meaning; relationships with family and friends and colleagues get twisted out of shape or destroyed. What dying persons need, therefore, can range from relatively simple (clysis for maintaining hydration when a patient can't drink, for example) to enormously complex (helping a patient making the decision to be removed from a respirator). Coping with dying patients' changing needs as they move along that spectrum demands enormous creativity and flexibility on the part of everyone involved with their care. Fortunately, end-of-life care has begun to emerge as a meaningful discipline in its own right; a new and very large "black bag" containing a wide variety of techniques and treatments is becoming available to help with the hard work of dying.[7]

Anyone who has cared for a significant number of dying patients recognizes that a small proportion of terminally ill patients at some point move to the far end of the spectrum of needs. As a consequence, these patients decide that the work of staying alive has become too difficult to handle; that, despite the best that caregivers have to offer, life as they are experiencing it is no longer an acceptable option. In any other situation in which patients are seen to be suffering from the burden of illness, the medical imperative to caregivers is clear: make every reasonable effort to ease the burden. Unfortunately, when an unremitting and unmanageable terminal illness leads patients to the extreme decision that continued life is unacceptable, the options for caregivers are few, and difficult.

This is, of course, the very situation in which extreme measures become a consideration, including terminal sedation (which some consider extreme) or, if all else fails, assisted suicide. Viewed in the context of the spectrum of terminal illness, these measures lose some of their strangeness, since they can now be seen as simply representing appropriate care at the extreme end of the more familiar, overall spectrum of patients' needs. As such, they can be seen as entirely consistent with the fundamental task of medicine: the relief of suffering. But physicians are uncomfortable about using these interventions, for a variety of powerful reasons—legal, moral, spiritual. At a more practical level, doctors may simply feel trapped by the lack of acceptable alternatives, hence coerced into considering the use of extreme measures, and doctors hate, above all things, to feel coerced.

What are the alternatives in such situations? One is to continue to treat with the best interventions available, short of extreme measures, despite the recognition that those interventions are not helping to provide the patient with a peaceful death. This approach is seen by many as inhumane and as a denial of the validity of the patient's decision to end his or her life, hence a violation of patient autonomy. Another alternative is to remove oneself from the patient's care and let someone else (another physician, the patient, or the patient's family) handle the situation. To some physicians this approach amounts to abandonment; it is therefore likely to be repugnant to many physicians and their patients, particularly when they have had a long-standing relationship. The choices faced by physicians in such situations are excruciating.[8]

Ethics Aside, What's Wrong with Assisted Suicide?

Terminal illness obviously involves the feelings and experience of others, but dying belongs to the patient; no one can do it for them. Suicide, however, directly affects others besides the person who has died, in ways that can be uniquely damaging. For one thing, suicide is particularly damaging precisely because the suicide's death was self-inflicted. Those closest to the person who has committed suicide invariably feel particularly guilty ("if only I had done more, he wouldn't have killed himself . . . " or "sometimes I wished she was dead, and now it's happened . . . ") and angry ("he betrayed me: he chose to leave me . . . "). The intensity and quality of feeling frequently go well beyond those associated with all deaths, and this legacy is made even more bitter because there is no chance for forgiveness. In addition to its professional, ethical, spiritual, and legal difficulties, assisted suicide therefore carries with it an added burden, one that is not often considered: a serious and lasting social and emotional price among the survivors.

Summing Up

Twenty years ago, in my small practice of about 300 patients, a patient dying of a malignancy asked me to write him a large prescription for barbiturates to keep in case he decided he could no longer tolerate living with his illness. At no point in my medical school training and residency had anyone ever introduced the subject; never had I encountered a discussion of the issues in the nonmedical media; and it had never come up previously in my practice. I told my patient I couldn't do it.

In the hospital where I trained as a resident, the chief of medicine did not hesitate to remind us that a patient's decision to sign out against medical advice was really our problem. Thinking back on it, therefore, I suppose I reacted to my patient's request for barbiturates the way I did partly because I felt that if he had to ask, it was my problem: I hadn't been doing my job as a doctor properly. I think I would probably feel largely the same way today. On the other hand, the topic of assisted suicide is no longer taboo. In the past five to ten years the topic has been widely aired and in fact has become an object of enormous interest, analysis, and debate, both scholarly and popular, involving not only people in medicine but dying patients and their families. All of that seems to me to be to the good; as medical professionals, we are no longer operating quite so idiosyncratically in this area, making decisions in isolation, feeling our way along in the dark.

Perhaps the most important lesson we have learned from all of this is that unlike our previous way of viewing it, it is a mistake to see assisted suicide in terms of absolutes. Assisted suicide looks different, depending on where you sit (or lie). We have also learned that the work of dying is hard. Given that reality, we should not be surprised if, when suffering is extreme despite the best that palliative care has to offer, the work of dying can on occasion become too much for a patient to manage.

We can't be shocked or surprised, therefore, if in such situations assisted suicide seems to the patient, and sometimes to the patient's family as well, both logical and desirable. Indeed, it may seem to them the only acceptable way for a patient to maintain dignity and control, and to achieve at least a somewhat peaceful death. We can't be shocked or surprised if, in those circumstances, patients sometimes ask us for help in dying. And if, as some doctors are convinced, the medical imperative is always to relieve patients' suffering, we also can't be shocked or surprised when some doctors agree to assist the rare patient with ending a life that has become, irreversibly and intractably, intolerable.[9] Legal issues aside, the absolute condition for such a decision is, of course, that both patient and doctor must agree that actively ending the patient's life has become the only acceptable means of ending such an extreme assault by disease on the patient's personhood.

On the other hand, by sharing the experiences of caring for dying patients more openly within the profession, we have also learned the extent to which the idea of assisting patients seems to violate individual doctors' deepest professional and personal codes. And we have learned the extent to which assisted suicide carries a uniquely heavy social and emotional cost, an important truth echoed in an old saying: "Take what you want, said the Lord—and pay."

All of these lessons are right—which leaves us in the uncomfortable position of living with an unresolved, and irresolvable, tension. In my view, that's exactly where we should be. The only real tragedy would be if we were to become comfortable with the choices we face in caring for patients whose illness has made the work of living—and dying—intolerable.

REFERENCES

1. S. B. Nuland, *How We Die: Reflections on Life's Final Chapter* (New York: Knopf, 1994).
2. E. Becker, *The Denial of Death* (New York: Free Press, 1973); and A.D. Weisman, *On Dying and Denying: A Psychiatric Study of Terminality* (New York: Behavioral Publications, 1972).
3. F. Davidoff, "Who Has Seen a Blood Sugar? The Shaping of the Invisible World," in *Who Has Seen a Blood Sugar? Reflections on Medical Education* (Philadelphia: American College of Physicians, 1996), 96–100.
4. S. Sontag, *Illness as Metaphor* (New York; Farrar, Straus, and Giroux, 1978).
5. A. T. Carron, J. Lynn, and P. Keaney, "End-of-Life Care in Medical Textbooks," *Annals of Internal Medicine* 130 (1999): 82–86.
6. E. J. Cassell, *The Nature of Suffering and the Goals of Medicine* (New York: Oxford University Press, 1991).
7. B. Lo, L. Snyder, and H. C. Sox, "Care at the End of Life: Guiding Practice Where There Are No Easy Answers," *Annals of Internal Medicine* 130 (1999): 772–774.
8. W. J. Kade, "Death with Dignity: A Case Study," *Annals of Internal Medicine* 132 (2000): 504–506.
9. E. J. Emanuel et al., "Attitudes and Practices of U.S. Oncologists regarding Euthanasia and Physician-Assisted Suicide," *Annals of Internal Medicine* 133 (2000): 527–532.

Assisted Suicide:
An Annotated Bibliography

PETER N. POON, J.D., M.A.

Consensus Statements

S. Heilig et al., "Physician-Hastened Death: Advisory Guidelines for the San Francisco Bay Area from the Bay Area Network of Ethics Committees," *Western Journal of Medicine* 166 (1997): 370–378.

In 1996 the Bay Area Network of Ethics Committees (BANEC) convened to draft practice guidelines for physician-assisted suicide. Members included experts in medicine, oncology, hospice care, and ethics. Complete consensus on the guidelines was rare, with "majority rule" being the deciding factor. The guidelines were envisioned for usage by individuals and health care institutions in the local area should physician-assisted suicide become legal. Among other points, the final guidelines state the following: Patients requesting physician-assisted suicide should be referred to hospice or a palliative care expert; no physician or other health care worker is required to participate in an assisted suicide; the patient should have a terminal diagnosis, be mentally competent, and have decision-making capability; palliative care should be made accessible to the patient; a second opinion should be sought; the patient should sign a witness consent form; the physician or designated person should be available until the patient's death; and a registry should track all cases of physician-assisted suicide.

New York State Task Force on Life and the Law, *When Death Is Sought: Assisted Suicide and Euthanasia in the Medical Context* (Albany: New York State Task Force, 1994).

The twenty-five members of this task force—physicians, nurses, lawyers, academics, and religious representatives—held different views about the ethical acceptability of assisted suicide. Nonetheless, the task force unanimously recommended that the state law prohibiting assisted suicide and euthanasia *not* be changed. The group drew a clear line between forgoing medical interventions (allowable) and physician-assisted suicide. Legalizing physician-assisted suicide would be "profoundly dangerous" to large segments of the population, according to the task force, especially given the current failure of many physicians to treat pain and depression adequately. The task force agreed that the provision of pain medication to alleviate pain is ethically acceptable even if such treatment may hasten the patient's death. Professional standards of conduct should be guided by the legal prohibition against assisted suicide.

"Physician-Assisted Suicide: Toward a Comprehensive Understanding. Report of the Task Force on Physician-Assisted Suicide of the Society for Health and Human Values," *Academic Medicine* 70 (1995): 583–590.

In 1992 the Society for Health and Human Values (SHHV) created a task force to deliberate on the issue of physician-assisted suicide. Rather than formulating definitive positions on the issue, the resulting document discusses a number of topics and questions from various perspectives. The topics are as follows: the moral status of suicide, clinical and epidemiological aspects of suicide, the relevance of voluntary choice, the nature of professional duty, and social implications. These topics generated questions such as, What different approaches are used to assess the morality of suicide; what empirical assumptions are made about suicide that reflect value choices; what are the scope and limits of respect for patient autonomy; should family members have veto power over a patient's physician-assisted suicide request; what does a physician's professional duty encompass; how will a particular stance on physician-assisted suicide affect patient trust; and what are the slippery slopes associated with legalizing physician-assisted suicide? The SHHV report concludes with a number of questions for patients to consider when contemplating assisted suicide.

E. W. Young et al., "Report of the Northern California Conference for Guidelines on Aid-in-Dying: Definitions, Differences, Convergences, Conclusions," *Western Journal of Medicine* 166 (1997): 381–388.

In 1996 the Stanford University Center for Biomedical Ethics convened a conference to develop guidelines on physician-assisted suicide. The 108 participants included ethics committee members, academic medicine, health lawyers, aging experts, physicians, and religious representatives, among others. Various working groups made the following conclusions, although minority opinions were sometimes expressed: Only patients with an incurable condition causing intolerable, irremediable suffering, who voluntarily request physician-assisted suicide, should be eligible for it (terminal illness is not a requirement); access to adequate palliative care is a prerequisite; decisional capacity is required, and a mental health evaluation should be performed if there is any doubt; families should be involved in but not have veto power over patients' decisions; physicians should be free to not participate in assisted suicide; guidelines should be devised to minimize potential hazards of physician-assisted suicide in the managed care context; ethics committees should have an advisory role in physician-assisted suicide; and institutional participation in physician-assisted suicide requires debate and consensus building at many institutional levels.

K. Haley and M. Lee, eds., *The Oregon Death with Dignity Act: A Guidebook for Health Care Providers* (Portland: Oregon Health Sciences University, 1998).

L. Snyder and A. L. Caplan, eds., "Assisted Suicide: Finding Common Ground," *Annals of Internal Medicine* 132 (2000): 468–499.

Clinical Guidelines

C. H. Coleman and A. R. Fleischman, "Guidelines for Physician-Assisted Suicide: Can the Challenge Be Met?" *Journal of Law, Medicine, and Ethics* 24 (1996): 217–224.

This article compares and contrasts several proposed guidelines for implementing physician-assisted suicide should it be legalized; namely, the "Quill Guidelines" (1992), the "Miller Guidelines" (1994), and the "Model Act" (1996). The authors oppose legalization of physician-assisted suicide because none of these guidelines are likely to limit assisted suicide to narrowly defined circumstances. They raise two concerns: the slippery-slope problem (physician-assisted suicide will be used for a broader set of circumstances than intended), and physicians' inability to determine whether the criteria would have been met, even if there are certain, circumscribed cases in which physician-assisted suicide would be ethically defensible. According to the authors, the proposed guidelines fail to offer a realistic mechanism for monitoring the practice of physician-assisted suicide.

M. A. Drickamer, M. A. Lee, and L. Ganzini, "Practical Issues in Physician Assisted Suicide," *Annals of Internal Medicine* 126 (1997): 146–151.

This article approaches the issue of physician-assisted suicide by assuming its legalization, then exploring the practical skills that physicians would need to know in order to assist in a patient's death. These skills would include an understanding of patients' motivations for requesting physician-assisted suicide, assessing mental status, diagnosing and treating depression, maximizing palliative interventions, and evaluating any external pressures on the patient. Physicians will be expected to prognosticate about life expectancy and the onset of functional and cognitive decline, and to provide information about effective medications and dosages. Patient confidentiality would have to be balanced against the need of health care professionals and institutions to access patient information. Physicians would also have to be knowledgeable about insurance coverage and managed care options related to physician-assisted suicide. Each of these issues is explored in depth in this article.

L. L. Emanuel, "Facing Requests for Physician-Assisted Suicide: Toward a Practical and Principled Clinical Skill Set," *Journal of the American Medical Association* 280 (1998): 643–647.

An eight-step approach for responding to physician-assisted suicide requests is offered in this article. This approach relies solely on two well-accepted principles: Patients should be free of unwanted interventions, and physicians are obligated to provide comfort care to suffering patients. At any step along the way, if the patient drops the physician-assisted suicide request, care should be provided as discussed previously with the patient/proxy. If the patient continues to request physician-assisted suicide, the clinician should progress to the next step. The eight steps are: (1) evaluate for depression, (2) assess decision-making capacity, (3) undergo advance care planning, (4) establish and treat root causes of physician-assisted suicide request, (5) provide full information about alternatives, (6) consult with professional colleagues, (7) review adherence to goals and care plan, and (8) if request continues, decline physician-assisted suicide but provide care as discussed. While this approach never includes physician-assisted suicide as an option, it does allow for removal of unwanted life-support interventions and opioid or anesthetic coma for patients in unrelievable pain.

T. E. Quill, C. K. Cassell, and D. E. Meier, "Care of the Hopelessly Ill: Proposed Clinical Criteria for Physician-Assisted Suicide," *New England Journal of Medicine* 327 (1992): 1380–1384.

The authors support legalizing physician-assisted suicide but not active euthanasia because of the risk of abuse that the latter practice would entail. However, the authors believe that physician-assisted suicide may be appropriate when incurably ill patients suffer intolerably despite comprehensive efforts to provide palliative care. Seven clinical criteria are proposed: (1) the patient's condition is incurable and associated with severe, unrelenting suffering; the illness does not have to be terminal, however; (2) the patient's suffering and request for physician-assisted suicide are not because of inadequate comfort care; (3) the patient clearly, repeatedly, and freely initiates a request to die; (4) the patient's judgment is not distorted, by depression for example; (5) physician-assisted suicide is carried out in the context of a meaningful patient-physician relationship; (6) another experienced physician is consulted; and (7) the physician-assisted suicide is clearly documented. Additionally, the authors suggest that close family members should be part of the decision-making process and that the physician should be present at the patient's death.

A. L. Caplan, L. Snyder, and K. Faber-Langendoen, "The Role of Guidelines in the Practice of Physician-Assisted Suicide," *Annals of Internal Medicine* 132 (2000): 476–481.

K. Faber-Langendoen and J. H. T. Karlawish, "Should Assisted Suicide Be Only Physician Assisted? *Annals of Internal Medicine* 132 (2000): 482–487.

K. M. Foley, "The Relationship of Pain and Symptom Management to Patient Requests for Physician-Assisted Suicide," *Journal of Pain and Symptom Management* 6 (1991): 289–297.

S. Miles, D. M. Pappas, and R. Koepp, "Considerations of Safeguards Proposed in Laws and Guidelines to Legalize Assisted Suicide," in *Physician-Assisted Suicide*, ed. R. F. Weir (Bloomington: Indiana University Press, 1997), 205–223.

S. G. Post, "Physician-Assisted Suicide in Alzheimer's Disease," *Journal of the American Geriatrics Society* 45 (1997): 647–651.

L. R. Slome et al., "Physician-Assisted Suicide and Patients with Human Immunodeficiency Virus Disease," *New England Journal of Medicine* 336 (1997): 417–421.

J. A. Tulsky, R. Ciampa, and E. J. Rosen, "Responding to Legal Requests for Assistance in Dying," *Annals of Internal Medicine* 132 (2000): 494–499.

Empirical Data and Attitudinal Surveys

D. A. Asch, "The Role of Critical Care Nurses in Euthanasia and Assisted Suicide," *New England Journal of Medicine* 334 (1996): 1374–1379.

Compiling the responses of 852 critical care nurses in the United States, this report found that 17 percent of the nurses had received requests from patients or family members to perform euthanasia or to assist in a suicide, and 16 percent had engaged in such practices. On average, each nurse complied with 8 percent of the requests from patients and 12 percent of the requests from surrogates. Five percent of the nurses who reported performing euthanasia or assisted suicide had done so more than twenty times. It was estimated that 5 percent of nurses had engaged in euthanasia or assisted suicide without a request from either the patient or a surrogate, and 8 percent had done so without a request from the attending physician. A weakness of the study was that it did not distinguish between euthanasia and assisted suicide (the questionnaire gave examples of euthanasia but not of assisted suicide). Recurring themes were found in the respondents' written comments: the overuse of life-sustaining technology, a sense of responsibility for the patient's welfare, a desire to relieve suffering, and a desire to overcome the perceived unresponsiveness of physicians toward suffering.

E. J. Emanuel et al., "The Practice of Euthanasia and Physician-Assisted Suicide in the United States: Adherence to Proposed Safeguards and Effects on Physicians," *Journal of the American Medical Association* 280 (1998): 507–513.

In a recent effort to describe the practice of euthanasia and physician-assisted suicide in the United States, Emanuel and colleagues interviewed 355 randomly selected oncologists, using a method modeled on the Remmelink study in the Netherlands. Fifty-six (15.8 percent) of the respondents reported participating in euthanasia or physician-assisted suicide. Based on a subset of the respondents, the authors found that 15.8 percent of patients did not participate in the decision for euthanasia or physician-assisted suicide, 97.4 percent of patients were experiencing unremitting pain or such poor physical functioning they could not perform self-care, and physicians sought consultation in 39.5 percent of cases. Moreover, 23.7 percent of physicians regretted having performed euthanasia or assisted suicide.

H. Koenig, D. Wildman-Hanlon, and K. Schmader, "Attitudes of Elderly Patients and Their Families toward Physician-Assisted Suicide," *Archives of Internal Medicine* 156 (1996): 2240–2248.

In a survey of elderly patients with medical and psychiatric problems and their family members, 39.9 percent of the patients held a favorable attitude toward physician-assisted suicide in cases of terminal illness, while 59.3 percent of the relatives held a favorable attitude. Moreover, the relatives demonstrated only a marginal ability to predict patients' attitudes toward physician-assisted suicide. Neither spouses nor adult children were consistently better at predicting patients' attitudes, and agreement between relatives was poor. Citing other studies, the authors aver that more vulnerable patients such as the elderly express significantly less favor toward physician-assisted suicide than less vulnerable populations do. Relatives' marginal ability to predict patients' attitudes toward physician-assisted suicide is cause for concern when substituted judgment is used in the case of demented patients.

R. Mangus, A. Dipeiro, and C. Hawkins, "Medical Students' Attitudes toward Physician-Assisted Suicide," *Journal of the American Medical Association* 282 (1999): 2080–2081.

This study compares the attitudes toward physician-assisted suicide as reported by medical students in Oregon (where the practice is legal) and U.S. medical students (fourth year only) outside of Oregon. Both study groups favored the legalization of physician-assisted suicide at similar rates (64 percent and 66 percent, respectively). However, when asked about willingness to write a lethal prescription, only 52 percent of the Oregon students expressed such willingness, compared with 60 percent of the control (non-Oregon) group. Moreover, when the responses of fourth-year Oregon students were isolated, only 44 percent expressed willingness to prescribe lethal medication. The authors posit that the added emphasis on alternative approaches to end-of-life care in Oregon's medical curriculum might lead fourth-year students to believe that compliance with a physician-assisted suicide request is unnecessary.

D. E. Meier et al., "A National Survey of Physician-Assisted Suicide and Euthanasia in the United States," *New England Journal of Medicine* 338 (1998): 1193–1201.

Based on approximately 1,900 completed questionnaires, Meier and colleagues found that 11 percent of physicians (from the ten specialties most likely to receive requests for assisted suicide or euthanasia) responded that they would be willing to hasten a patient's death by prescribing medication under current legal constraints. An additional 7 percent said that they would provide a lethal injection. If physician-assisted suicide were made legal, the willingness to engage in it increased to 36 percent. Eighteen percent of physicians reported actually having received a request for assisted suicide; 16 percent of these physicians wrote at least one prescription to hasten death, and 59 percent of the patients used the prescriptions to end their lives. Perceived reasons for patients' requests for physician-assisted suicide or euthanasia included discomfort other than pain (79 percent), loss of dignity (53 percent), fear of uncontrollable symptoms (52 percent), actual pain (50 percent), loss of meaning in their lives (47 percent), being a burden (34 percent), and dependency (30 percent). Nineteen percent of patients who received a prescription for a lethal dose of medication were clinically depressed. Interestingly, only 3 percent of patients who received physician-assisted suicide were female.

D. P. Sulmasy et al., "Physician Resource Use and Willingness to Participate in Assisted Suicide," *Archives of Internal Medicine* 158 (1998): 974–978.

Because of the suggestion that cost control measures might have a deleterious effect on end-of-life decision making, Sulmasy and colleagues investigated whether a correlation exists between physicians' tendency to conserve medical resources and their willingness to participate in physician-assisted suicide. Using a hypothetical of a competent terminally ill patient with breast cancer who makes stable and persistent requests for physician-assisted suicide, 33 percent of the survey respondents (general internists) indicated that they would participate in the hypothetical patient's suicide. Those who were more conservative with resources were 6.4 times more likely to prescribe the lethal dose of drugs than those who were considered resource-intensive. Although a strong, linear relationship between resource use and willingness to participate in assisted suicide was established, the authors admit that other causal factors might be present (e.g., risk aversion).

D. L. Willems, E. R. Daniels, and E. J. Emanuel, "Attitudes and Practices concerning the End of Life: A Comparison between Physicians from the United States and from the Netherlands," *Archives of Internal Medicine* 160 (2000): 63–68.

One hundred fifty-two physicians from Oregon (prior to implementation of the Oregon Death with Dignity Act) and sixty-seven physicians from the Netherlands were interviewed using the same questions about physician-assisted suicide and other end-of-life issues. A similar proportion of Oregonian and Dutch physicians endorsed physician-assisted suicide (53 percent and 56 percent, respectively), although the former are significantly more likely to provide physician-assisted suicide when the patient's main concern is about burdening his or her family (24 percent versus 9 percent). The authors hypothesize that differences in the valuation of autonomy and differences in systems of health care coverage may explain this difference in attitude. Forty-five percent of the physicians from Netherlands have performed either physician-assisted suicide or euthanasia, compared with 7 percent of the Oregon physicians. Dutch physicians viewed euthanasia and physician-assisted suicide as ethically acceptable in equal proportions, while physicians from Oregon were consistently less likely to find euthanasia acceptable as compared to physician-assisted suicide.

B. J. Daly et al., "Thoughts of Hastening Death among Hospice Patients," *Journal of Clinical Ethics* 11 (2000): 56–65.

L. Ganzini et al., "Attitudes of Patients with Amyotrophic Lateral Sclerosis and Their Care Givers toward Assisted Suicide," *New England Journal of Medicine* 339 (1998): 967–973.

P. Phillips, "Views of Assisted Suicide from Several Nations," *Journal of the American Medical Association* 278 (1997): 969–970.

T. E. Quill et al., "The Debate over Physician-Assisted Suicide: Empirical Data and Convergent Views," *Annals of Internal Medicine* 128 (1998): 553–558.

L. W. Roberts et al., "Internal Medicine, Psychiatry, and Emergency Medicine Residents' Views of Assisted Death Practices," *Archives of Internal Medicine* 157 (1997): 1603–1609.

V. P. Tilden et al., "Oregon's Physician-Assisted Suicide Vote: Its Effect on Palliative Care," *Nursing Outlook* 44 (1996): 80–83.

J. Wolfe et al., "Stability of Attitudes regarding Physician-Assisted Suicide and Euthanasia among Oncology Patients, Physicians, and the General Public," *Journal of Clinical Oncology* 17 (1999): 1274–1279.

Cases

T. E. Quill, "Doctor, I Want to Die. Will You Help Me?" *Journal of the American Medical Association* 270 (1993): 870–873.

Quill reports on a number of cases in which a patient requests assistance in dying from his or her physician. The statement, "Doctor, I want to die," and the question, "Will you help me?" must be separately understood and explored. The wish to die can have potential meanings: weariness from acute medical treatment; unrecognized or undertreated physical symptoms; emergent psychosocial problems; spiritual crisis; clinical depression; or unrelenting, intolerable suffering. When faced with a request for help in dying, physicians should consider the following recommendations: listen to the patient, be compassionate and caring, promise to not abandon the patient, be honest about one's position on physician-assisted suicide, try to approach intolerable suffering with an open mind, and maintain one's own support systems.

L. Snyder and J. Weiner, "Physician-Assisted Suicide," in *Ethical Choices: Case Studies for Medical Practice*, ed. L Snyder (Philadelphia: American College of Physicians, 1996).

A case of a sixty-year-old woman with pancreatic cancer who requests physician-assisted suicide is explored. "Ella Washington" probably has less than six months to live, clearly understands her condition, and has a supportive family. She fears a painful, lingering death, dependence, and disability, and she wants to "die with dignity." After a psychiatric consult verifies that she is not significantly depressed, her doctor writes a prescription for barbiturates. The case commentary notes that most patients find that high-quality hospice-type care meets their needs, but a few like Mrs. Washington desire more control. Relevant issues are then debated, such as conflicting goods (preservation of life, restoration of health, relief of suffering, respect for patient autonomy), sanctity of life, and slippery slopes.

S. W. Tolle and L. Snyder, "Physician-Assisted Suicide Revisited: Comfort and Care at the End of Life," in *Ethical Choices*, ed. Snyder.

A fifty-year-old man with metastatic adenocarcinoma is the subject of this case study. Mr. Jensen decides to forgo recommended surgery and, moreover, asks his doctor to increase the morphine concentration in his self-administered pump so that he can take his own life. His sons support this action, but his wife, whom he has appointed as his surrogate decision-maker, is ambivalent. The hospice nurses find assisted suicide to be morally objectionable. The commentary on this case states that the initial response to a request for assisted suicide should be further conversation to determine the patient's unmet needs, fears, suffering, social circumstances, and pain. Pain relief and treatment of depression must be emphasized and properly administered. The moral conscience of involved health care providers should be respected, and family members' burdens should be considered.

P. A. Ubel, "Assisted Suicide and the Case of Dr. Quill and Diane," *Issues in Law and Medicine* 8 (1993): 487–502.

Hospice and Palliative Care

W. G. Bartholome, "Physician-Assisted Suicide, Hospice, and Rituals of Withdrawal," *Journal of Law, Medicine, and Ethics* 24 (1996): 233–236.

In reviewing the federal Circuit Courts' 1996 opinions on physician-assisted suicide (*Compassion in Dying v. State of Washington* and *Quill v. Vacco*), the author characterizes as a glaring omission the courts' failure to discuss hospice care as an alternative to physician-assisted suicide. The hospice philosophy counters our society's view of life and death, which is shaped by professionals and technology, rationality, and a desire for control and by a problem-solving mentality. The author, himself diagnosed with a terminal illness, advocates adopting a "ritual of withdrawal." He describes what he imagines his withdrawal ritual will be like as he nears death, which includes a loving spouse, a supportive family, and a home in which to die.

A. L. Caplan, "Will Assisted Suicide Kill Hospice?" in *Ethics in Hospice Care: Challenges to Hospice Values in a Changing Health Care Environment*, ed. B. Jennings (New York: Haworth Press, 1997), 17–24.

The hospice movement has traditionally emphasized the importance of maintaining quality of life during the process of dying and has spurned assisting patients in committing suicide. Caplan holds that the increasing support for assisted suicide will change the way in which hospice works or is used. Instead of personal self-determination, a value that hospice supports, the debate surrounding assisted suicide is more about fear, guilt, cost, and dignity according to Caplan. He views hospice as unable to address these quality-of-life and "suffering" concerns adequately. Moreover, he predicts that in the future, assisted suicide will not be restricted to the terminally ill, the population with which hospice is solely concerned. If hospice is to endure, it must provide a convincing argument as to why its vision of dying is more attractive and affordable than assisted suicide.

K. M. Foley, "Competent Care for the Dying Instead of Physician-Assisted Suicide" (editorial), *New England Journal of Medicine* 336 (1997): 54–59.

In this editorial Foley argues that the federal Circuit Courts' assertions of a constitutional right to assisted suicide (*Compassion in Dying v. State of Washington* and *Quill v. Vacco*) may further devalue the lives of terminally ill patients and may allow society to abrogate its responsibility for their care. She opines that the Circuit Courts' rejection of a distinction between "letting die" and "killing" runs counter to medical standards. Withdrawal of treatment followed by palliative care respects patients' autonomous decisions not to be battered by medical technology. Unlike physician-assisted suicide, however, the physician's intent is to provide care, not death. Foley cites data to support a number of assertions: The desire for death is closely associated with depression, with pain and lack of social support as contributing factors; physicians are inadequately trained in palliative care of the dying; and vulnerable patients receive less pain treatment than do other groups of patients. Legalizing physician-assisted suicide, according to the author, would result in its practice becoming a substitute for interventions that might otherwise enhance the quality of life for dying patients.

I. R. Byock, "Consciously Walking the Fine Line: Thoughts on a Hospice Response to Assisted Suicide and Euthanasia," *Journal of Palliative Care* 9 (1993): 25–28.
J. Loconte, "Hospice, Not Hemlock: The Medical and Moral Rebuke to Doctor-Assisted Suicide," *Policy Review* 88 (1998): 40–48.
T. E. Quill, B.C. Lee, and S. Nunn, "Palliative Treatments of Last Resort: Choosing the Least Harmful Alternative," *Annals of Internal Medicine* 132 (2000): 488–493.
R. L. Worsnop, "Caring for the Dying: Would Better Palliative Care Reduce Support for Assisted Suicide?" *CQ Researcher* 7, no. 33 (1997): 771–791.

Constitutional Issues

R. Bopp and J. E. Colson, "Three Strikes: Is an Assisted Suicide Right Out?" *Issues in Law and Medicine* 15 (1999): 3–86.

This article suggests that the United States Supreme Court's rejection of a constitutional right to assisted suicide in *Washington v. Glucksberg,* 117 S.Ct. 2258 (1997) and *Vacco v. Quill,* 117 S.Ct. 2293 (1997) was the first major strike against the movement to legalize physician-assisted suicide. The second strike was the Florida Supreme Court's decision, which found no state constitutional right to physician-assisted suicide (*Krischer v. McIver,* 697 So.2d 97 [Fla. 1997]). Other state supreme courts are likely to follow Florida's suit, according to the authors. The third strike has been the repeated rejection of state legislative efforts to legalize assisted suicide. While these three strikes have stemmed the movement to legalize physician-assisted suicide, the authors warn that ballot initiatives have the potential to reverse this trend. They conclude that federal statutory or constitutional protection is needed to block the legalization of physician-assisted suicide. This article offers an in-depth legal analysis of the preceding points, with particular attention to the U.S. Supreme Court's recent rulings.

Y. Kamisar, "On the Meaning and Impact of the Physician-Assisted Suicide Cases," *Minnesota Law Review* 82 (1998): 895–922.

Kamisar reviews the U.S. Supreme Court's decisions in *Washington v. Glucksberg* and *Vacco v. Quill,* intending to demonstrate the magnitude of the setback for proponents of physician-assisted suicide. These proponents have attempted to characterize the decisions as a judicial "green light" for legislative legalization of physician-assisted suicide. However, Kamisar points out that legislatures have always had the "green light" to legalize physician-assisted suicide. In fact, none of the state legislative bills to legalize it have passed, while sixteen bills to prohibit assisted suicide have been enacted. The author then indicates how the U.S. Supreme Court disagreed with the lower federal courts on four principal points, ruling that (1) the distinction between assisting suicide and terminating lifesaving treatment is widely recognized in the medical and legal tradition; (2) the law distinguishes actions taken "because of" a given end from actions taken "in spite of" their unintended but foreseen consequences (principle of double effect); (3) *Cruzan* is not a precedential assisted suicide case but, rather, was based on the traditional right to bodily integrity and freedom from unwanted touching; and (4) the broad language in *Casey* about "choices central to personal dignity and autonomy" did not suggest that all intimate and personal decisions such as assistance in dying are constitutionally protected. Kamisar also provides a lengthy rationale on why Justice Sandra Day O'Connor's concurring opinions in *Glucksberg* and *Quill* do not signal a possible right to physician-assisted suicide in compelling circumstances.

D. Orentlicher, "The Supreme Court and Physician-Assisted Suicide: Rejecting Assisted Suicide but Embracing Euthanasia," *New England Journal of Medicine* 337 (1997): 1236–1239.

This article reviews the U.S. Supreme Court's recent decisions rejecting a constitutional right to physician-assisted suicide (*Washington v. Glucksberg* and *Vacco v. Quill*). While the Court seems to have upheld the distinction between withdrawal of life-sustaining treatment and assisted suicide or euthanasia, the article argues that the Court in fact undermined the distinction when it endorsed the practice of terminal sedation. The author contends that terminal sedation is often a form of euthanasia. In many cases, the terminally sedated patient dies from a combination of two intentional acts by the physician: induction of unconsciousness and withholding of food and water. The latter act cannot be justified under the principle of double effect, according to the author, because it only serves to bring about the patient's death. He concludes that physician-assisted suicide is ethically better than terminal sedation.

G. J. Annas, "The Bell Tolls for a Constitutional Right to Physician-Assisted Suicide," *New England Journal of Medicine* 337 (1997): 1098–1103.
R. Burt, "Disorder in the Court: Physician-Assisted Suicide and the Constitution," *Minnesota Law Review* 82 (1998): 965–981.
S. M. Canick, "Constitutional Aspects of Physician-Assisted Suicide after *Lee v. Oregon*," *American Journal of Law and Medicine* 23 (1997): 69–96.
J. E. Linville, "Physician-Assisted Suicide as a Constitutional Right," *Journal of Law, Medicine, and Ethics* 24 (1996): 198–206.

Legalization

A. M. Capron, "Legalizing Physician-Aided Death," *Cambridge Quarterly of Healthcare Ethics* 5 (1996): 10–23.

Capron examines the question of whether society ought to recognize, as a matter of positive law, an individual's right to physician-assisted suicide. In arguing against its legalization, he raises a number of policy considerations: the likelihood of prognostic mistakes (e.g., predicting time of death); the ineffectiveness of consultation requirements if the consulting physician is not independent of the attending physician; no guarantee that the patient is acting voluntarily and competently at the time of suicide (but only when the prescription is written); and the slippery slope to euthanasia or the extension of a right to physician-assisted suicide to non-terminally ill patients, minors, and so on (assisted suicide on demand).

F. G. Miller, H. Brody, and T. E. Quill, "Can Physician-Assisted Suicide Be Regulated Effectively?" *Journal of Law, Medicine, and Ethics* 24 (1996): 225–232.

Miller, Brody, and Quill respond to a number of objections to their 1994 proposed regulatory scheme for physician-assisted suicide. Among other safeguards, their proposal requires the physician to consult with another independent physician skilled in palliative care who must determine that all of the policy criteria and requirements have been satisfied; this consultant would report to a regional palliative care committee. The authors contend that physicians will comply with the legal requirements even though some physicians flout the current prohibitions against physician-assisted suicide. The authors concede that the confidentiality of physician-patient interactions risks inappropriate use of physician-assisted suicide and that "regulation necessarily depends on a degree of trust in the professional integrity of physicians." The authors also respond to other objections to their regulatory scheme such as the implications of unequal access to

health care in the United States, the managed care environment, resistance to oversight and bureaucratic interference, and the inadequate availability of palliative care consultants. They characterize the
proposed regulation as a hypothesis and are willing to take the risk
of being mistaken.

D. Orentlicher, "The Legalization of Physician-Assisted Suicide: A Very Modest
Revolution," *Boston College Law Review* 38 (1997): 443–475.

Published just one month before the U.S. Supreme Court's decisions
in *Washington v. Glucksberg* and *Vacco v. Quill,* this law review article
posited that the legal distinction between withdrawal of life-sustaining
treatment and physician-assisted suicide has eroded. That conclusion was premature given the Court's subsequent rulings (see Orentlicher, "The Supreme Court and Physician-Assisted Suicide"). Relying
heavily on the Ninth and Second Circuit opinions that recognized a
constitutional right to assisted suicide (overturned by the Supreme
Court), Orentlicher argues that there is no moral distinction between
assisted suicide and treatment withdrawal and that the traditional legal distinction was a mere proxy for the public sentiment which condoned treatment withdrawal but not assisted suicide. He further contends that the increasing recognition of a right to assisted suicide
indicates that the proxy role has become outdated and that the underlying moral concern is with the patient's condition (i.e., terminal
illness) rather than whether death comes by treatment withdrawal or
suicide. Finally, Orentlicher predicts that the right to die will further
expand to include assisted suicide for non-terminally ill patients
and/or euthanasia.

C. H. Baron et al., "A Model State Act to Authorize and Regulate Physician-
Assisted Suicide," *Harvard Journal on Legislation* 33 (1996): 1–34.
E. J. Emanuel, "What Is the Great Benefit of Legalizing Euthanasia or Physician-
Assisted Suicide? Symposium on Physician-Assisted Suicide," *Ethics* 109
(1999): 629–642.
F. G. Miller, "Legalizing Physician-Assisted Suicide by Judicial Decision: A Criti-
cal Appraisal," *BioLaw* (July–August 1996): S136–S145.
J. Schwartz, "Writing the Rules of Death: State Regulation of Physician-Assisted
Suicide," *Journal of Law, Medicine, and Ethics* 24 (1996): 207–216.

Discrimination

A. I. Batavia, "Disability and Physician-Assisted Suicide," *New England Journal
of Medicine* 336 (1997): 1671–1673.

In this article the author supports a right to physician-assisted suicide
despite arguments about potential discrimination against persons
with disabilities. He cites a Harris poll which found that 66 percent
of people with disabilities supported a right to assisted suicide (as

compared with 70 percent of the general population). Opponents of physician-assisted suicide argue that persons with disabilities will be coerced into choosing it if it is legalized. The author, however, counters that the disability-rights movement is founded on the right to self-determination, which should include control over the timing and manner of imminent death from a terminal illness. While a system of physician-assisted suicide may result in some individual cases of discrimination, this imperfection is not adequate justification for denying autonomy to persons in the terminal stage of illness according to the author. The issue is whether regulatory safeguards can be effective and whether the risks of abuse outweigh the individual's rights of autonomy and privacy.

A. Silvers, "Protecting the Innocents from Physician-Assisted Suicide: Disability Discrimination and the Duty to Protect Otherwise Vulnerable Groups," in *Physician Assisted Suicide: Expanding the Debate*, ed. M. P. Battin, R. Rhodes, and A. Silvers (New York: Routledge, 1998), 133–148.

This article criticizes the stereotype of persons with disabilities as incompetent, easily coerced, and inclined to end their lives. The author argues that a fine line separates a benign disposition and a malignantly paternalistic one. Characterizing a class of persons as weak deprives them of the power of self-determination. By winning recognition of his/her competence to control his/her own dying, the person with a disability gains control over his or her life. Substituting public judgment about the well-being of people with disabilities over their own personal assessments is disrespectful according to the author. Finally, the author argues that illness and disability are conceptually different, and persons with disabilities should not be consigned to the "sick role."

R. L. Burgdorff, "Assisted Suicide: A Disability Perspective," *Issues in Law and Medicine* 14 (1998): 273–300.
K. L. Kirschner, C. J. Gill, and C. K. Cassel, "Physician-Assisted Suicide in the Context of Disability," in *Physician-Assisted Suicide*, ed. Weir, 155–66.
M. C. Siegel, "Legal Pity: The Oregon Death with Dignity Act, Its Implications for the Disabled, and the Struggle for Equality in an Able-Bodied World," *Law and Inequality* 16 (1998): 259–288.

The Oregon Act

A. E. Chin et al., "Legalized Physician-Assisted Suicide in Oregon: The First Year's Experience," *New England Journal of Medicine* 340 (1999): 577–583.

On 27 October 1997 physician-assisted suicide became legal under the Oregon Death with Dignity Act. Stringent guidelines on the manner and scope of physician-assisted suicides were set forth in the act. Chin and colleagues report on the effects of the law in its first year of operation. They examined all of the available data on Oregon residents who received prescriptions for lethal medications under the Oregon act and compared them with persons who died from similar illnesses in the same year but who did not receive such prescriptions. Twenty-three persons received prescriptions for lethal medications; fifteen died from the medications (5 of every 10,000 deaths in Oregon in 1998), six died from underlying illnesses, and two were still alive as of 1 January 1999. Thirteen of the fifteen who died after physician-assisted suicide had cancer. The case patients and controls were similar with regard to sex, race, urban or rural residence, level of education, health insurance coverage, and hospice enrollment. None of the patients expressed concern about the financial impact of their illness, and only one case patient expressed concern about inadequate control of pain at the end of life. However, case patients were significantly more likely than control patients were to have expressed concern about loss of autonomy and loss of bodily function control. Persons who were divorced or had never married were more likely than married persons were to choose physician-assisted suicide. The median duration of the patient-physician relationship was 69 days for case patients, compared with 720 days for control patients.

K. Foley and H. Hendin, "The Oregon Report: Don't Ask, Don't Tell," *Hastings Center Report* 29 (1999): 37–42.

The authors, who opposed passage of Oregon's Death with Dignity Act, issue a critique of the Oregon Health Division's report on the first year's experience under the act. This article questions the basis for the report's conclusion that assisted suicide is being carried out safely under the statute. Specifically, the authors contend that the report failed to assess the physical, psychological, and existential needs of the patients requesting assisted suicide. For example, the report concluded that economic factors did not influence the choice of assisted suicide based on the fact that none of the patients expressed financial concerns to their physicians. Physicians, however, are not required under the act to inquire about patients' economic or social circumstances. Other examples are given to support a case of flawed monitoring and unwarranted conclusions.

L. Ganzini et al., "Physicians' Experiences with the Oregon Death with Dignity Act," *New England Journal of Medicine* 342 (2000): 557–563.

This recent report describes the level and details of legalized physician-assisted suicide in the state of Oregon. Of the 2,649 physician respondents, 221 requests for prescriptions for lethal medications were recorded since enactment of the Oregon Death with Dignity Act in 1997. About one in six prescription requests were granted, but only one in ten of the requests actually resulted in suicide. Physicians implemented at least one substantive palliative intervention for sixty-eight patients. Of those who received palliative intervention, 46 percent changed their minds about assisted suicide. By comparison, only 15 percent of those for whom no substantive interventions were made changed their minds.

A.D. Sullivan, K. Hedberg, and D. W. Fleming, "Legalized Physician-Assisted Suicide in Oregon—The Second Year," *New England Journal of Medicine* 342 (2000): 598–604.

This report describes the effects of Oregon's Death with Dignity Act in its second year of operation. In addition to information culled from physicians' reports, death certificates, and physician interviews, family members were also interviewed. In 1999, thirty-three persons received prescriptions for lethal medications. Twenty-seven individuals (9 per 10,000 deaths in Oregon) died after taking the medication (including one patient who received a prescription in 1998 but died in 1999), five died from underlying illnesses, and two were alive as of 1 January 2000. Seventeen of the twenty-seven patients who died after physician-assisted suicide had cancer. All twenty-seven patients had health insurance, 78 percent were receiving hospice care, 22 percent were widowed, 30 percent were divorced, and 4 percent were never married. Each interviewed family member knew of the patient's request for and use of lethal medication. The median interval between the first request for physician-assisted suicide and death was eighty-three days. Twenty-two physicians prescribed lethal medications in 1999; six of these physicians had also prescribed such medication in 1998. The most frequently cited reasons for requesting physician-assisted suicide were loss of autonomy (81 percent) and an inability to participate in activities that make life enjoyable (81 percent), although 26 percent included inadequate pain control as a concern. None of the patients reported the cost of treatment or prolonging life as a concern.

P. Curran, "Regulating Death: Oregon's Death with Dignity Act and the Legalization of Physician-Assisted Suicide," *Georgetown Law Journal* 86 (1998): 725–749.

E. J. Emanuel and E. Daniels, "Oregon's Physician-Assisted Suicide Law: Provisions and Problems," *Archives of Internal Medicine* 156 (1996): 825–829.

H. Hendin, K. Foley, and M. White, "Physician-Assisted Suicide: Reflections on Oregon's First Case," *Issues in Law and Medicine* 14 (1998): 243–270.

H. Wineberg, "Oregon's Death with Dignity Act: Fourteen Months and Counting," *Archives of Internal Medicine* 160 (2000): 21–25.

The Netherlands

J. H. Groenewoud et al., "Clinical Problems with the Performance of Euthanasia and Physician-Assisted Suicide in the Netherlands," *New England Journal of Medicine* 342 (2000): 551–556.

In this recent study, researchers analyzed data from two studies of euthanasia and physician-assisted suicide in the Netherlands, where physicians are not prosecuted if the act has been carried out under strict conditions. The researchers identified and categorized clinical problems in physician-assisted suicide and euthanasia cases as either technical problems (e.g., difficulty inserting an intravenous line), complications (e.g., myoclonus or vomiting), or problems with completion (e.g., longer-than-expected interval between administration of medications and death). Technical problems occurred in 10 percent of physician-assisted suicide cases, complications occurred in 7 percent of cases, and problems with completion occurred in 15 percent of cases. In 18 percent of cases of *intended* physician-assisted suicide, the physician ended up administering a lethal medication to the patient (resulting in euthanasia). In twelve of these cases, there had been problems with completion, and in five cases the patient had been unable to take all of the medications.

J. M. Cuperus-Bosma et al., "Assessment of Physician-Assisted Death by Members of the Public Prosecution in the Netherlands," *Journal of Medical Ethics* 25 (1999): 8–15.
H. Hendin, C. Rutenfrans, and Z. Zylicz, "Physician-Assisted Suicide and Euthanasia in the Netherlands: Lessons from the Dutch," *Journal of the American Medical Association* 277 (1997): 1720–1722.
G. van der Wal et al., "Evaluation of the Notification Procedure for Physician-Assisted Death in the Netherlands," *New England Journal of Medicine* 335 (1996): 1706–1711.

Moral Arguments For and Against Assisted Suicide

M. Battin and L. Snyder, "Should Older Persons Have the Right to Commit Suicide?" in *Controversial Issues in Aging,* ed. A. E. Scharlach and L. W. Kaye (Boston: Allyn Bacon, 1996), 92–102.

Battin and Snyder take opposite positions on the question of whether older persons should have the right to commit suicide. Battin argues for such a right by proposing a simple syllogism: Older persons should have the right to shape the character of their own life in accord with their own basic values; shaping the character of one's own life includes shaping the process of dying; thus, older persons should have the right to shape the process of dying. Battin states (but does not defend) that the premises of this syllogism are uncontroversial and that while the conclusion is controversial, it should not be. She views suicide as a fundamental right and holds that suicide in old age may represent a considered, principled choice. Snyder counters that the purposes and consequences of self-determination must be examined for both the individual and society. Rights have limits and corresponding responsibilities. Whereas the right to protect oneself from bodily invasion is generally accepted, a "right" to suicide represents a *positive* right that must concede to some limits. The integrity of the medical profession is one such consideration that must be accounted for in asserting a right to assisted suicide.

D. W. Brock, "Physician-Assisted Suicide Is Sometimes Morally Justified," in *Physician-Assisted Suicide*, ed. Weir, 86–103.

This chapter lays out the moral claim that physician-assisted suicide (and euthanasia) is morally justified in certain individual cases. Brock appeals to the same ethical values that support patients' rights to withhold or withdraw life-sustaining treatment: individual self-determination or autonomy and individual well-being. He admits that physician-assisted suicide and euthanasia constitute deliberate killing but insists that not every deliberate killing in the practice of medicine is morally impermissible. To support this conclusion, he relies on the notion that forgoing life-sustaining treatment (which is commonly accepted as morally permissible) is not "allowing to die" but, rather, killing. A physician who allows or enables a patient to forgo or withdraw life-sustaining treatment acts in a manner intended to cause death, does in fact cause death, and therefore kills. Thus, at least some deliberate killings are permissible in medicine. A killing is wrongful, according to Brock, when it deprives a person of a great good: the patient's future and future plans. When a competent individual no longer finds continued life a good, or finds the means of preserving it unacceptable, it is morally justifiable for him or her to reject life-sustaining treatment and likewise to request assistance in committing suicide. Under a rights approach to the morality of killing, a competent person may waive the right not to be killed if continued life is not wanted.

D. Callahan, "Physician-Assisted Suicide: Moral Questions," in *End-of-Life Decisions: A Psychosocial Perspective*, ed. M. D. Steinberg and S. J. Youngner (Washington: American Psychiatric Press, 1998), 283–297.

Callahan challenges the basic claims supporting the legalization of physician-assisted suicide, namely, the right to self-determination and the obligation (especially of physicians) to relieve suffering. Beyond the duty to relieve suffering, there is another obligation: knowing when suffering cannot or should not be wholly overcome. Suffering may sometimes exist so that some other human good can be accomplished. Physicians have a duty to respond to the psychological suffering of illness but not to a deeper level of suffering that entails the meaning of life and fundamental philosophical and religious questions. Medicine is not competent to address the meaning of life and death, only the physical and psychological manifestations of those problems. On a separate point, Callahan argues that the requirements of mental competence and suffering/terminal illness are two separate requirements which physician-assisted suicide proponents have arbitrarily joined. Each requirement should stand as an independent justification for physician-assisted suicide, yet proponents are reluctant to separate the two, thus demonstrating the weakness of their position.

M. Gunderson, "A Right to Suicide Does Not Entail a Right to Assisted Death," *Journal of Medical Ethics* 23 (1997): 51–54.

For the purposes of this piece, the author assumes without argument that it is permissible for a person to commit suicide, and that people have a right to commit suicide. However, he argues that the permissibility of assistance in suicide and a right to such assistance do not follow from the prior assumptions. Rather, the prior assumptions only establish a right not to have unreasonable restrictions placed on the means by which one can exercise one's right to commit suicide. Whether a restriction, such as a prohibition against physician-assisted suicide, is reasonable depends on policy considerations. Does a proposed regulation (e.g., prohibiting physician-assisted suicide) violate the core of the right to commit suicide? One must determine what value the right to commit suicide protects, and whether the benefits gained by the use of suicide assistance are overridden by harmful consequences.

E. D. Pellegrino, "Doctors Must Not Kill," *Journal of Clinical Ethics* 3 (1992): 95–102.

In this article Pellegrino extends his arguments against active euthanasia to encompass physician-assisted suicide. First, he rebuts a number of moral arguments that have been made in support of euthanasia/physician-assisted suicide by distinguishing between killing and letting die, disputing that euthanasia/physician-assisted suicide promotes patient autonomy, arguing that beneficence does not require killing because inevitable suffering may serve some purposes, and rejecting the necessity of euthanasia given available palliative care measures. Next, Pellegrino asserts that the practice of euthanasia and physician-assisted suicide would seriously distort the healing foundation of the patient-physician relationship. Physician-assisted suicide would shake patients' trust in their physicians and would seriously affect the physician's own psyche. Finally, Pellegrino posits that euthanasia/physician-assisted suicide would lead to grave social consequences, using a slippery-slope line of reasoning.

T. Salem, "Physician-Assisted Suicide: Promoting Autonomy—or Medicalizing Suicide?" *Hastings Center Report* 29 (1999): 30–36.

A unique perspective on physician-assisted suicide is offered in this article. The author argues that physician-assisted suicide does not demedicalize death as many of its proponents suppose but, rather, medicalizes suicide. Suicide is moved from the private arena to medicine's stewardship when physicians' assistance is involved. Physician-assisted suicide effects the medicalization of suicide as an act, as a practice, and as a moral and social ethos. Second, physician-assisted suicide is an impediment to, rather than a facilitator of, individual autonomy. Even proponents of physician-assisted suicide insist on certain safeguards in order to ensure the "voluntariness" of the act. This implies that someone other than the patient has greater expertise in judging the appropriateness of the request. The medical establishment is given the authority to make these judgments and thus to curtail the patient's autonomy. The author points out that the medicalization of suicide may not be reconcilable with patient autonomy.

J. Jarvis Thomson, "Physician-Assisted Suicide: Two Moral Arguments, Symposium on Physician-Assisted Suicide," *Ethics* 109 (1999): 497–518.

Two moral arguments against the legalization of physician-assisted suicide are considered then rebutted in this article. The first argument against physician-assisted suicide makes a distinction between killing and letting a patient die; the former is always morally impermissible while the latter is permissible in some circumstances. The author counters that the prohibition against killing doesn't "hit all of its target" because it does not apply to physician-assisted suicide (the doctor herself does not kill the patient). Moreover, the killing/letting die distinction "hits what it should not hit": Providing a lethal dose of morphine as the only way to relieve a patient's pain constitutes a killing, yet it is considered morally permissible. The second argument against physician-assisted suicide states that a physician's action that intends to cause a patient's death is morally different from an action in which death is merely foreseen. The former is always morally impermissible while the latter is permissible in some circumstances (the principle of double effect). The author rebuts this distinction by proffering counterexamples that attempt to undermine the utility and persuasiveness of the principle of double effect.

Y. Kamisar, "The Reasons So Many People Support Physician-Assisted Suicide —and Why These Reasons Are Not Convincing," *Issues in Law and Medicine* 12 (1996): 113–131.

F. G. Miller, "A Communitarian Approach to Physician-Assisted Death," *Cambridge Quarterly of Healthcare Ethics* 6 (1997): 78–87.

S. M. Wolf, "Gender, Feminism, and Death: Physician-Assisted Suicide and Euthanasia," in *Feminism and Bioethics: Beyond Reproduction*, ed. S. M. Wolf (New York: Oxford University Press, 1996), 287–317.

Causation, Double Effect, Alternatives, and Distinctions

F. G. Miller and D. E. Meier, "Voluntary Death: A Comparison of Terminal Dehydration and Physician-Assisted Suicide," *Annals of Internal Medicine* 128 (1998): 559–562.

> The authors propose terminal dehydration as a morally more acceptable alternative to physician-assisted suicide in most cases. Terminal dehydration, or voluntarily forgoing food and water, respects self-determination, is accessible to any suffering patient able to make decisions, preserves professional integrity because it does not require physicians to provide the means of death, and does not require a change in law or public policy because patients have a legal and moral right to refuse medical treatment, including food and water. Evidence indicates that terminal dehydration is not painful, and any physical discomfort can be alleviated by standard palliative measures. On the other hand, unlike physician-assisted suicide, death is not swift. Death normally occurs in several days, but in some cases, it takes up to three or four weeks. The emotional toll on family members may be high. During this period, patients may be vulnerable to outside pressure to change their minds. The authors offer some clinical advice on effecting terminal dehydration: The patient's decision must be informed and voluntary, antidepressant therapy or counseling may be appropriate, the initiation of terminal dehydration should come from the patient, clinicians should continue to provide palliative care, and patients should be assured that they will not be abandoned.

T. E. Quill, B. Lo, and D. Brock, "Palliative Options of Last Resort: A Comparison of Voluntarily Stopping Eating and Drinking, Terminal Sedation, Physician-Assisted Suicide, and Voluntary Active Euthanasia," *Journal of the American Medical Association* 278 (1997): 2099–2104.

> Four means of hastening death are compared: voluntarily stopping eating and drinking, terminal sedation, physician-assisted suicide, and voluntary active euthanasia. The article first defines each practice and compares their clinical and legal status. An ethical comparison of the four practices is the heart of this article. The authors argue that the doctrine of double effect and the active/passive distinction are not useful philosophical tools for determining the ethical acceptability of the different practices. Rather, the patient's wishes and competent consent are more ethically relevant. The authors also emphasize the importance of proportionality; i.e., the greater the patient's suffering, the greater risk the physician can take in potentially contributing to the patient's death. Finally, the article lists five categories of safeguards that should be adhered to for any of the four methods

of hastening death: palliative care; informed consent; diagnostics and prognostic clarity; independent second opinion; and document and review.

D. Sulmasy, "Killing and Allowing to Die: Another Look," *Journal of Law, Medicine, and Ethics* 26 (1998): 55–64.

In its decision rejecting a constitutional right to physician-assisted suicide, the U.S. Supreme Court upheld the distinction between killing patients and allowing them to die. Nevertheless, a number of persons (including the Second Circuit Court of Appeals) have argued against making this distinction. Sulmasy explicates the traditional distinction between killing and allowing to die in a clear fashion, supporting the long tradition it has held in medicine and in common morality. After carefully defining the terms "killing" and "allowing to die," he states the traditional view as follows: "Except in cases of self-defense or rescue, *all* Killing* is morally wrong. *Some* Allowing to Die* is also morally wrong, and some is not." Next, Sulmasy describes the role of intention. Intention is different from belief and desire; intention involves commitment. In killing, intentions are uniform (to achieve death); in allowing to die, the intentions vary. Where the clinician's intention in allowing a patient to die is the death of the patient, such allowances are morally wrong. The article also includes discussions about recognizing intentions, public policy, and why intending death is wrong.

H. Brody, "Causing, Intending, and Assisting Death," *Journal of Clinical Ethics* 4 (1993): 112–117.
T. Cavanaugh, "Currently Accepted Practices That Are Known to Lead to Death, and PAS: Is There an Ethically Relevant Difference?" *Cambridge Quarterly of Healthcare Ethics* 7 (1998): 375–382.
J. Deigh, "Physician-Assisted Suicide and Voluntary Euthanasia: Some Relevant Differences," *Journal of Criminal Law and Criminology* 88 (1998): 1155–1165.
F. G. Miller, J. J. Fins, and L. Snyder, "Assisted Suicide Compared with Refusal of Treatment: A Valid Distinction?" *Annals of Internal Medicine* 132 (2000): 470–475.

Professional Integrity

S. H. Miles, "Physician-Assisted Suicide and the Profession's Gyrocompass," *Hastings Center Report* 25 (1995): 17–19.

In this piece Miles advocates a professional ethic that counterbalances the prevailing trend toward autonomy-based ethics. He decries the "medicalization" of suicide, which characterizes the act of suicide as a medical judgment rather than an existential one. Suicide is a socio-personal event, not a medicopersonal event. Professional integrity can be preserved where a physician assists in the suicide of a patient with whom he or she has an intimate relationship, or where the patient is suffering intractably. However, professional integrity is compromised when public policy explicitly grants physicians the right or exclusive authority to assist in patients' suicides. Aiding a suffering patient to commit suicide may be seen as an exceptional event which is consistent with professional integrity, but publicly providing prospective permission to engage in physician-assisted suicide would be detrimental to the profession of medicine.

F. G. Miller and H. Brody, "Professional Integrity and Physician-Assisted Death," *Hastings Center Report* 25 (1995): 8–17.

In this piece, it is proposed that physician-assisted suicide in exceptional cases may be consistent with professional integrity. Professional integrity is said to encompass the values, norms, and virtues that are distinctive and characteristic of physicians. The hallmarks of physician integrity are practicing competently, benefiting patients and avoiding harm, refraining from misrepresentation, and preserving patients' trust. The authors argue that each of these characteristics can be preserved in the case of physician-assisted suicide. For example, they reason that death should not always be regarded as a harm and that removing the evil of unrelievable suffering is a benefit, even if the benefit cannot be experienced. The authors also posit that physician-assisted suicide can be consistent with the goals of medicine, i.e., healing, promoting health, and helping patients achieve a peaceful and dignified death. While the authors conclude that physician-assisted suicide does not necessarily violate professional integrity, they admit that other moral considerations besides professional integrity may be appealed to in favor of, or against, permitting physician-assisted suicide.

M. P. Battin, "Is a Physician Ever Obligated to Help a Patient Die?" in *Regulating How We Die*, ed. Emanuel, 21–47, 264–267.
I. R. Byock, "Physician-Assisted Suicide Is *Not* an Acceptable Practice for Physicians," in *Physician-Assisted Suicide*, ed. Weir, 107–135.
R. Momeyer, "Does Physician Assisted Suicide Violate the Integrity of Medicine?" *Journal of Medicine and Philosophy* 20 (1995): 13–24.
T. E. Quill and C. K. Cassel, "Nonabandonment: A Central Obligation for Physicians," *Annals of Internal Medicine* 122 (1995): 368–374.
D. C. Thomasma, "When Physicians Choose to Participate in the Death of Their Patients: Ethics and Physician-Assisted Suicide," *Journal of Law, Medicine, and Ethics* 24 (1996): 183–197.

Religious Viewpoints

J. F. Childress, "Religious Viewpoints," in *Regulating How We Die*, ed. Emanuel, 294–300.

Childress focuses on the Judaic, Roman Catholic, and Protestant faiths as they bear on the issue of assisted suicide. These religions all believe in God's sovereignty and control over life and death, and they generally oppose assisted suicide based on religious-moral arguments against suicide itself. Human beings, created in God's image, have a negative obligation to refrain from killing themselves or others. Roman Catholicism stresses that we are not owners of our lives. However, a distinction is made between direct and indirect killing based on the rule of double effect. Moreover, acceptance of physical suffering is commended as a way of responding to tests of God, although such suffering is not necessarily obligatory. Protestantism is more individualistic about life-and-death decisions. The Anglican tradition appears to condone some instances of killing if the good outweighs the evil and cannot be achieved in a less destructive manner. Jewish tradition holds that an "unwillful" suicide excuses the agent, and most suicides are treated as unwillful. Childress is careful to note that for each of these religious traditions, differences in the structure and authority of particular religious organizations are relevant, not all participants in a particular religious community accept its official positions, and religious communities often recognize a difference between moral responses and pastoral responses to acts such as suicide or assisted suicide.

C. L. H. Traina, "Religious Perspectives on Assisted Suicide," *Journal of Criminal Law and Criminology* 88 (1998): 1147–1154.

All of the major religious traditions, according to this article, have a history of opposition to physician-assisted suicide. Maintaining the process of dying as a natural one stems from the belief that one's final hours are profoundly significant for reincarnation, afterlife, or resurrection. For most Jews who do not believe in an afterlife, the prohibition against assisted suicide is based on the concept that one should not trespass the divine prerogative to determine the moment of death. Muslims emphasize that all suffering has a divine purpose. Two notable exceptions in the Protestant religion are the Unitarian Universalist Association and the liberal portions of the United Church of Christ, which provide some support for those who choose physician-assisted suicide. The author opines that assisted suicide is not ultimately a matter of religious freedom, however. The critical query is whether physician-assisted suicide erodes or sustains the values and rights to which we are socially and constitutionally committed. Finally, the author offers a feminist perspective that opposes the legalization of physician-assisted suicide.

E. N. Dorff, "Assisted Death: A Jewish Perspective," in *Must We Suffer Our Way to Death? Cultural and Theological Perspectives on Death by Choice,* ed. R. P. Hamel and E. R. DuBose (Dallas: Southern Methodist University Press, 1996), 141–173.

H. T. Engelhardt, "Physician-Assisted Suicide Reconsidered: Dying as a Christian in a Post-Christian Age," *Christian Bioethics* 4 (1998): 143–167.

P. B. Jung, "Dying Well Isn't Easy: Thoughts of a Roman Catholic Theologian on Assisted Death, in *Must We Suffer Our Way to Death?,* ed. Hamel and DuBose, 174–197.

J. J. Paris and M. P. Moreland, "A Catholic Perspective on Physician-Assisted Suicide," in *Physician Assisted Suicide: Expanding the Debate,* ed. M. P. Battin, R. Rhodes, and A. Silvers (New York: Routledge, 1998), 324–333.

A. Verhey, "Assisted Suicide and Euthanasia: A Biblical and Reformed Perspective, in *Must We Suffer Our Way to Death?,* ed. Hamel and DuBose, 226–265.

Public Policy

E. Emanuel, "The Future of Euthanasia and Physician-Assisted Suicide: Beyond Rights Talk to Informed Public Policy," *Minnesota Law Review* 82 (1998): 983–1014.

The U.S. Supreme Court's decision in *Washington v. Glucksberg* and *Vacco v. Quill* changes the physician-assisted suicide debate from one about rights to one about public policy, according to this article. Although some of the justices left open the possibility that a more limited constitutional right to physician-assisted suicide might later be found, the author argues that the factual predicates of these possibly protected instances of physician-assisted suicide are so unlikely to occur that such a narrow constitutional right will never be declared. In analyzing Justice Stephen Breyer's suggestion that a "right to die with dignity" might be recognized, the author posits that the perceived "dignity" associated with physician-assisted suicide is in reality the social sanction conferred by professional medical assistance; death is "medicalized" or aesthetically sanitized. The proper forum for debating whether physician-assisted suicide should be socially sanctioned is the legislature, not the courts. In furthering this debate, the author argues that the "typical" picture of a painful dying process painted by physician-assisted suicide advocates is a myth. He also contends that the potential harms of legalizing physician-assisted suicide would outweigh the benefits. He attempts to quantify both benefits and harms, but ultimately his estimations remain speculative.

J. A. Tulsky, A. Alpers, and B. Lo, "A Middle Ground on Physician-Assisted Suicide," *Cambridge Quarterly of Healthcare Ethics* 5 (1996): 33–43.

The authors of this article claim to take a middle ground on physician-assisted suicide by proposing that statutes prohibiting physician-assisted suicide be amended such that physicians can assert an exonerating affirmative defense when certain criteria are met. The defendant would bear the burden of proof in asserting the following defense: "An act otherwise constituting criminal assistance to suicide is not punishable if the defendant proves by clear and convincing evidence that the suicidal individual was a competent adult who was suffering from an incurable terminal disease, that the individual suffered physical distress despite appropriate supportive care, and that the suicidal action was voluntary." The authors believe that such an affirmative defense would bring the law into accord with society's values and practice, that it would diminish the likelihood of prosecution, and that it would stimulate discussion of physician-assisted suicide without violating the patient's privacy.

S. M. Wolf, "Physician-Assisted Suicide in the Context of Managed Care," *Duquesne Law Review* 35 (1996): 455–480.

This law review examines the potential effect of managed care on the practice of physician-assisted suicide if legalized. The author concludes that physicians practicing under managed care may have strong financial incentives to perform assisted suicide since it would likely be less costly than alternatives such as aggressive treatment or a palliative care regimen. Especially at risk under managed care's cost containment schemes would be vulnerable populations such as the elderly and the poor. She also argues that managed care would further drive patients to request assisted suicide because of systemic neglect; studies show that managed care organizations have a relatively poor record in responding to depression. Based on the above, the author criticizes the Ninth Circuit Court's decision in *Compassion in Dying v. Washington,* 79 F.3d 790 (9th Cir. 1996), for relying on outdated assumptions about physician behavior and the patient-physician relationship. Constitutional analysis should account for the realities of the current health care system, which is dominated by managed care.

J. C. d'Oronzio, "Rappelling on the Slippery Slope: Negotiating Public Policy for Physician-Assisted Death," *Cambridge Quarterly of Healthcare Ethics* 6 (1997): 113–117.
C. A. Tauer, "Philosophical Debate and Public Policy on Physician-Assisted Death," in *Must We Suffer Our Way to Death?,* ed. Hamel and DuBose, 45–65.

M. Teitelman, "Not in the House: Arguments for a Policy of Excluding Physician-Assisted Suicide from the Practice of Hospital Medicine," in *Physician Assisted Suicide*, ed. Battin et al., 203–222.

W. J. Winslade, "Physician-Assisted Suicide: Evolving Public Policies," in *Physician-Assisted Suicide*, ed. Weir, 224–239.

APPENDIX B

The Oregon Death with Dignity Act

OREGON REVISED STATUTES, 1996
SUPPLEMENT S127.800—127.897

SECTION ONE: General Provisions

1.01 DEFINITIONS

The following words and phrases, whenever used in this Act, shall have the following meanings:

(1) "Adult" means an individual who is 18 years of age or older.

(2) "Attending physician" means the physician who has primary responsibility for the care of the patient and treatment of the patient's disease.

(3) "Consulting physician" means the physician who is qualified by specialty or experience to make a professional diagnosis and prognosis regarding the patient's disease.

(4) "Counseling" means a consultation between a state licensed psychiatrist or psychologist and a patient for the purpose of determining whether the patient is suffering from a psychiatric or psychological disorder, or depression causing impaired judgment.

(5) "Health care provider" means a person licensed, certified, or otherwise authorized or permitted by the law of this State to administer health care in the ordinary course of business or practice of a profession, and includes a health care facility.

(6) "Incapable" means that in the opinion of a court or in the opinion of the patient's attending physician or consulting physician, a patient lacks the ability to make and communicate health care decisions to health care providers, including communication through persons familiar with the patient's manner of communicating if those persons are available. Capable means not incapable.

(7) "Informed decision" means a decision by a qualified patient, to request and obtain a prescription to end his or her life in a humane and dignified manner, that is based on an appreciation of the relevant facts and after being fully informed by the attending physician of:

    (a) his or her medical diagnosis;

    (b) his or her prognosis;

    (c) the potential risks associated with taking the medication to be prescribed;

    (d) the probable result of taking the medication to be prescribed;

> (e) the feasible alternatives, including, but not limited to, comfort
> care, hospice care and pain control.

(8) "Medically confirmed" means the medical opinion of the attending physician has been confirmed by a consulting physician who has examined the patient and the patient's relevant medical records.

(9) "Patient" means a person who is under the care of a physician.

(10) "Physician" means a doctor of medicine or osteopathy licensed to practice medicine by the Board of Medical Examiners for the State of Oregon.

(11) "Qualified patient" means a capable adult who is a resident of Oregon and has satisfied the requirements of this Act in order to obtain a prescription for medication to end his or her life in a humane and dignified manner.

(12) "Terminal disease" means an incurable and irreversible disease that has been medically confirmed and will, within reasonable medical judgment, produce death within six (6) months.

SECTION TWO: Written Request for Medication to End One's Life in a Humane and Dignified Manner

2.01 WHO MAY INITIATE A WRITTEN REQUEST FOR MEDICATION

An adult who is capable, is a resident of Oregon, and has been determined by the attending physician and consulting physician to be suffering from a terminal disease, and who has voluntarily expressed his or her wish to die, may make a written request for medication for the purpose of ending his or her life in a humane and dignified manner in accordance with this Act.

2.02 FORM OF THE WRITTEN REQUEST

(1) A valid request for medication under this Act shall be in substantially the form described in Section 6 of this Act, signed and dated by the patient and witnessed by at least two individuals who, in the presence of the patient, attest that to the best of their knowledge and belief the patient is capable, acting voluntarily, and is not being coerced to sign the request.

(2) One of the witnesses shall be a person who is not:
> (a) A relative of the patient by blood, marriage or adoption;
> (b) A person who at the time the request is signed would be entitled to any portion of the estate of the qualified patient upon death under any will or by operation of law; or
> (c) An owner, operator or employee of a health care facility where the qualified patient is receiving medical treatment or is a resident.

(3) The patient's attending physician at the time the request is signed shall not be a witness.

(4) If the patient is a patient in a long term care facility at the time the written request is made, one of the witnesses shall be an individual designated by the facility and having the qualifications specified by the Department of Human Resources by rule.

SECTION THREE: Safeguards

3.01 ATTENDING PHYSICIAN RESPONSIBILITIES

The attending physician shall:

(1) Make the initial determination of whether a patient has a terminal disease, is capable, and has made the request voluntarily;

(2) Inform the patient of;
    (a) his or her medical diagnosis;
    (b) his or her prognosis;
    (c) the potential risks associated with taking the medication to be prescribed;
    (d) the probable result of taking the medication to be prescribed;
    (e) the feasible alternatives, including, but not limited to, comfort care, hospice care and pain control.

(3) Refer the patient to a consulting physician for medical confirmation of the diagnosis, and for determination that the patient is capable and acting voluntarily;

(4) Refer the patient for counseling if appropriate pursuant to Section 3.03;

(5) Request that the patient notify next of kin;

(6) Inform the patient that he or she has an opportunity to rescind the request at any time and in any manner, and offer the patient an opportunity to rescind at the end of the 15 day waiting period pursuant to Section 3.06;

(7) Verify, immediately prior to writing the prescription for medication under this Act, that the patient is making an informed decision;

(8) Fulfill the medical record documentation requirements of Section 3.09;

(9) Ensure that all appropriate steps are carried out in accordance with this Act prior to writing a prescription for medication to enable a qualified patient to end his or her life in a humane and dignified manner.

3.02 CONSULTING PHYSICIAN CONFIRMATION

Before a patient is qualified under this Act, a consulting physician shall examine the patient and his or her relevant medical records and confirm, in writing, the attending physician's diagnosis that the patient is suffering from a terminal disease, and verify that the patient is capable, is acting voluntarily and has made an informed decision.

3.03 COUNSELING REFERRAL

If in the opinion of the attending physician or the consulting physician a patient may be suffering from a psychiatric or psychological disorder, or depression causing impaired judgment, either physician shall refer the patient for counseling. No medication to end a patient's life in a humane and dignified manner shall be prescribed until the person performing the counseling determines that the person is not suffering from a psychiatric or psychological disorder, or depression causing impaired judgment.

3.04 INFORMED DECISION

No person shall receive a prescription for medication to end his or her life in a humane and dignified manner unless he or she has made an informed decision as defined in Section 1.01 (7). Immediately prior to writing a prescription for medication under this Act, the attending physician shall verify that the patient is making an informed decision.

3.05 FAMILY NOTIFICATION

The attending physician shall ask the patient to notify next of kin of his or her request for medication pursuant to this Act. A patient who declines or is unable to notify next of kin shall not have his or her request denied for that reason.

3.06 WRITTEN AND ORAL REQUESTS

In order to receive a prescription for medication to end his or her life in a humane and dignified manner, a qualified patient shall have made an oral request and a written request, and reiterate the oral request to his or her attending physician no less than fifteen (15) days after making the initial oral request. At the time the qualified patient makes his or her second oral request, the attending physician shall offer the patient an opportunity to rescind the request.

3.07 RIGHT TO RESCIND REQUEST

A patient may rescind his or her request at any time and in any manner without regard to his or her mental state. No prescription for medication under this Act may be written without the attending physician offering the qualified patient an opportunity to rescind the request.

3.08 WAITING PERIODS

No less than fifteen (15) days shall elapse between the patient's initial and oral request and the writing of a prescription under this Act. No less than 48 hours shall elapse between the patient's written request and the writing of a prescription under this Act.

3.09 MEDICAL RECORD DOCUMENTATION REQUIREMENTS

The following shall be documented or filed in the patient's medical record:
(1) All oral requests by a patient for medication to end his or her life in a humane and dignified manner;
(2) All written requests by a patient for medication to end his or her life in a humane and dignified manner;
(3) The attending physician's diagnosis and prognosis, determination that the patient is capable, acting voluntarily and has made an informed decision.
(4) The consulting physician's diagnosis and prognosis, and verification that the patient is capable, acting voluntarily and has made an informed decision;

(5) A report of the outcome and determinations made during counseling, of performed;

(6) The attending physician's offer to the patient to rescind his or her request at the time of the patient's second oral request pursuant to Section 3.06; and

(7) A note by the attending physician indicating that all requirements under this Act have been met and indicating the steps taken to carry out the request, including a notation of the medication prescribed.

3.10 RESIDENCY REQUIREMENTS

Only requests made by Oregon residents, under this Act, shall be granted.

3.11 REPORTING REQUIREMENTS

(1) The Health Division shall annually review a sample of records maintained pursuant to this Act.

(2) The Health Division shall make rules to facilitate the collection of information regarding compliance with this Act. The information collected shall not be a public record and may not be made available for inspection by the public.

(3) The Health Division shall generate and make available to the public an annual statistical report of information collected under Section 3.11(2) of this Act.

3.12 EFFECT ON CONSTRUCTION OF WILLS, CONTRACTS AND STATUTES

(1) No provision in a contract, will or other agreement, whether written or oral, to the extent the provision would affect whether a person may make or rescind a request for medication to end his or her life in a humane and dignified manner, shall be valid.

(2) No obligation owing under any currently existing contract shall be conditioned or affected by the making or rescinding of a request, by a person, for medication to end his or her life in a humane and dignified manner.

3.13 INSURANCE OR ANNUITY POLICIES

The sale, procurement, or issuance of any life, health, or accident insurance or annuity policy or the rate charged for any policy shall not be conditioned upon or affected by the making or rescinding of a request, by a person, for medication to end his or her life in a humane and dignified manner. Neither shall a qualified patient's act of ingesting medication to end his or her life in a humane and dignified manner have an effect upon a life, health, or accident insurance or annuity policy.

3.14 CONSTRUCTION OF ACT

Nothing in this Act shall be construed to authorize a physician or any other person to end a patient's life by lethal injection, mercy killing or active euthanasia. Actions taken in accordance with this Act shall not, for any purpose, constitute suicide, assisted suicide, mercy killing or homicide, under the law.

SECTION FOUR: Immunities and Liabilities

4.01 IMMUNITIES

Except as provided in Section 4.02:

(1) No person shall be subject to civil or criminal liability or professional disciplinary action for participating in good faith compliance with this Act. This includes being present when a qualified patient takes the prescribed medication to end his or her life in a humane and dignified manner.

(2) No professional organization or association, or health care provider, may subject a person to censure, discipline, suspension, loss of license, loss of privileges, loss of membership or other penalty for participating or refusing to participate in good faith compliance with this Act.

(3) No request by a patient for or provision by an attending physician of medication in good faith compliance with the provisions of this Act shall constitute neglect for any purpose of law or provide the sole basis for the appointment of a guardian or conservator.

(4) No health care provider shall be under any duty, whether by contract, by statute or by any other legal requirement to participate in the provision to a qualified patient of medication to end his or her life in a humane and dignified manner. If a health care provider is unable or unwilling to carry out a patient's health care provider shall transfer, upon request, a copy of the patient's relevant medical records to the new health care provider.

4.02 LIABILITIES

(1) A person who without authorization of the patient willfully alters or forges a request for medication or conceals or destroys a rescission of that request with the intent or effect of causing the patient's death shall be guilty of a Class A felony.

(2) A person who coerces or exerts undue influence on a patient to request medication for the purpose of ending the patient's life, or to destroy a rescission of such a request, shall be guilty of a Class A felony.

(3) Nothing in this Act limits further liability for civil damages resulting from other negligent conduct or intentional misconduct by any persons. (4) The penalties in this Act do not preclude criminal penalties applicable under other law for conduct which is inconsistent with the provisions of this Act.

SECTION FIVE: Severability

5.01 SEVERABILITY

Any section of this Act being held invalid as to any person or circumstance shall not affect the application of any other section of this Act which can be given full effect without the invalid section or application.

SECTION SIX: Form of the Request

6.01 FORM OF THE REQUEST

A request for a medication as authorized by this Act shall be in substantially the following form:

REQUEST FOR MEDICATION TO END MY LIFE IN A HUMANE AND DIGNIFIED MANNER

I, _____, am an adult of sound mind.

I am suffering from _____, which my attending physician has determined is a terminal disease and which has been medically confirmed by a consulting physician.

I have been fully informed of my diagnosis, prognosis, the nature of medication to be prescribed and potential associated risks, the expected result, and the feasible alternatives, including comfort care, hospice care and pain control.

I request that my attending physician prescribe medication that will end my life in a humane and dignified manner.

INITIAL ONE:

_____ I have informed my family of my decision and taken their opinions into consideration.

_____ I have decided not to inform my family of my decision.

_____ I have no family to inform of my decision.

> I understand that I have the right to rescind this request at any time.
> I understand the full import of this request and I expect to die when I take the medication to be prescribed.
> I make this request voluntarily and without reservation, and I accept full moral responsibility for my actions.

Signed: _____

Dated: _____

DECLARATION OF WITNESSES

We declare that the person signing this request:

(a) Is personally known to us or has provided proof of identity;
(b) Signed this request in our presence;
(c) Appears to be of sound mind and not under duress, fraud or undue influence;
(d) Is not a patient for whom either of us is attending physician.

_____ Witness 1/Date
_____ Witness 2/Date

Note: One witness shall not be a relative (by blood, marriage or adoption) of the person signing this request, shall not be entitled to any portion of the person's estate upon death and shall not own, operate or be employed at a health care facility where the person is a patient or resident. If the patient is an inpatient at a health care facility, one of the witnesses shall be an individual designated by the facility.

APPENDIX C

Supreme Court of the United States

SYLLABUS

WASHINGTON ET AL. V. GLUCKSBERG ET AL., 117 S.CT. 2258

ON WRIT OF CERTIORARI TO THE UNITED STATES COURT OF APPEALS
FOR THE NINTH CIRCUIT

No. 96-110

ARGUED JANUARY 8, 1997

DECIDED JUNE 26, 1997

It has always been a crime to assist a suicide in the State of Washington. The State's present law makes "promoting a suicide attempt" a felony, and provides: "A person is guilty of [that crime] when he knowingly causes or aids another person to attempt suicide." Respondents, four Washington physicians who occasionally treat terminally ill, suffering patients, declare that they would assist these patients in ending their lives if not for the State's assisted suicide ban. They, along with three gravely ill plaintiffs who have since died and a nonprofit organization that counsels people considering physician assisted suicide, filed this suit against petitioners, the State and its Attorney General, seeking a declaration that the ban is, on its face, unconstitutional. They assert a liberty interest protected by the Fourteenth Amendment's Due Process Clause which extends to a personal choice by a mentally competent, terminally ill adult to commit physician assisted suicide. Relying primarily on *Planned Parenthood of Southeastern Pa. v. Casey*, 505 U.S. 833, and *Cruzan v. Director, Mo. Dept. of Health*, 497 U.S. 261, the Federal District Court agreed, concluding that Washington's assisted suicide ban is unconstitutional because it places an undue burden on the exercise of that constitutionally protected liberty interest. The en banc Ninth Circuit affirmed.

Held: Washington's prohibition against "causing" or "aiding" a suicide does not violate the Due Process Clause. Pp. 5-32.

(a) An examination of our Nation's history, legal traditions, and practices demonstrates that Anglo American common law has punished or otherwise disapproved of assisting suicide for over 700 years; that rendering such assistance is still a crime in almost every State; that such prohibitions have never contained exceptions for those who were near death; that the prohibitions have in recent years been reexamined and, for the most part, reaffirmed in a number of States; and that the President recently signed the Federal Assisted Suicide Funding Restriction Act of 1997, which prohibits the use of federal funds in support of physician assisted suicide. Pp. 5-15.

(b) In light of that history, this Court's decisions lead to the conclusion that respondents' asserted "right" to assistance in committing suicide is not a fundamental liberty interest protected by the Due Process Clause. The Court's established method of substantive due process analysis has two primary features: First, the Court has regularly observed that the Clause specially protects those fundamental rights and liberties which are, objectively, deeply rooted in this Nation's history and tradition. *E.g., Moore* v. *East Cleveland,* 431 U.S. 494, 503 (plurality opinion). Second, the Court has required a "careful description" of the asserted fundamental liberty interest. *E.g., Reno* v. *Flores,* 507 U.S. 292, 302. The Ninth Circuit's and respondents' various descriptions of the interest here at stake—*e.g.,* a right to "determine the time and manner of one's death," the "right to die," a "liberty to choose how to die," a right to "control of one's final days," "the right to choose a humane, dignified death," and "the liberty to shape death"—run counter to that second requirement. Since the Washington statute prohibits "aiding another person to attempt suicide," the question before the Court is more properly characterized as whether the "liberty" specially protected by the Clause includes a right to commit suicide which itself includes a right to assistance in doing so. This asserted right has no place in our Nation's traditions, given the country's consistent, almost universal, and continuing rejection of the right, even for terminally ill, mentally competent adults. To hold for respondents, the Court would have to reverse centuries of legal doctrine and practice, and strike down the considered policy choice of almost every State. Respondents' contention that the asserted interest *is* consistent with this Court's substantive due process cases, if not with this Nation's history and practice, is unpersuasive. The constitutionally protected right to refuse lifesaving hydration and nutrition that was discussed in *Cruzan, supra,* at 279, was not simply deduced from abstract concepts of personal autonomy, but was instead grounded in the Nation's history and traditions, given the common law rule that forced medication was a battery, and the long legal tradition protecting the decision to refuse unwanted medical treatment. And although *Casey* recognized that many of the rights and liberties protected by the Due Process Clause sound in personal autonomy, 505 U.S., at 852, it does not follow that any and all important, intimate, and personal decisions are so protected, see *San Antonio School Dist.* v. *Rodriguez,* 411 U.S. 1, 33-34. *Casey* did not suggest otherwise. Pp. 15-24.

(c) The constitutional requirement that Washington's assisted suicide ban be rationally related to legitimate government interests, see *e.g., Heller* v. *Doe,* 509 U.S. 312, 319-320, is unquestionably met here. These interests include prohibiting intentional killing and preserving human life; preventing the serious public health problem of suicide, especially among the young, the elderly, and those suffering from untreated pain or from depression or other mental disorders; protecting the medical profession's integrity and ethics and maintaining physicians' role as their patients' healers; protecting the poor, the elderly, disabled persons, the terminally ill, and persons in other vulnerable groups from indifference, prejudice, and psychological and financial pressure to end their lives; and avoiding a possible slide towards voluntary and perhaps even involuntary euthanasia. The relative strengths of these various interests need not be weighed exactingly, since they are unquestionably important and legitimate, and the law at issue is at least reasonably related to their promotion and protection. Pp. 24-31.

79 F. 3d 790, reversed and remanded.

Rehnquist, C. J., delivered the opinion of the Court, in which O'Connor, Scalia, Kennedy, and Thomas, JJ., joined. O'Connor, J., filed a concurring opinion, in which Ginsburg and Breyer, JJ., joined in part. Stevens, J., Souter, J., Ginsburg, J., and Breyer, J., filed opinions concurring in the judgment.

Supreme Court of the United States

No. 96-110

WASHINGTON ET AL., PETITIONERS *v.* HAROLD GLUCKSBERG
ET AL.

ON WRIT OF CERTIORARI TO THE UNITED STATES COURT OF
APPEALS FOR THE NINTH CIRCUIT

[JUNE 26, 1997]

Chief Justice Rehnquist delivered the opinion of the Court.

The question presented in this case is whether Washington's prohibition against "causing" or "aiding" a suicide offends the Fourteenth Amendment to the United States Constitution. We hold that it does not.

It has always been a crime to assist a suicide in the State of Washington. In 1854, Washington's first Territorial Legislature outlawed "assisting another in the commission of self murder."[1] Today, Washington law provides: "A person is guilty of promoting a suicide attempt when he knowingly causes or aids another person to attempt suicide." Wash. Rev. Code 9A.36.060(1) (1994). "Promoting a suicide attempt" is a felony, punishable by up to five years' imprisonment and up to a $10,000 fine. §§9A.36.060(2) and 9A.20.021(1)(c). At the same time, Washington's Natural Death Act, enacted in 1979, states that the "withholding or withdrawal of life sustaining treatment" at a patient's direction "shall not, for any purpose, constitute a suicide." Wash. Rev. Code §70.122.070(1).[2]

Petitioners in this case are the State of Washington and its Attorney General.

Respondents Harold Glucksberg, M. D., Abigail Halperin, M. D., Thomas A. Preston, M. D., and Peter Shalit, M. D., are physicians who practice in Washington. These doctors occasionally treat terminally ill, suffering patients, and declare that they would assist these patients in ending their lives if not for Washington's assisted suicide ban.[3] In January 1994, respondents, along with three gravely ill, pseudonymous plaintiffs who have since died and Compassion in Dying, a nonprofit organization that counsels people considering physician assisted suicide, sued in the United States District Court, seeking a declaration that Wash Rev. Code 9A.36.060(1) (1994) is, on its face, unconstitutional. *Compassion in Dying* v. *Washington*, 850 F. Supp. 1454, 1459 (WD Wash. 1994).[4]

The plaintiffs asserted "the existence of a liberty interest protected by the Fourteenth Amendment which extends to a personal choice by a mentally competent, terminally ill adult to commit physician assisted suicide." *Id.*, at 1459. Relying primarily on *Planned Parenthood* v. *Casey*, 505 U.S. 833 (1992), and *Cruzan* v. *Director, Missouri Dept. of Health*, 497 U.S. 261 (1990), the District Court agreed, 850 F. Supp., at 1459-1462, and concluded that Washington's assisted suicide ban is unconstitutional because it "places an undue burden on the exercise of [that] constitutionally protected liberty interest." *Id.*, at 1465.[5] The District Court also decided that the Washington statute violated the Equal Protection Clause's requirement that "'all persons similarly situated . . . be treated alike.'" *Id.*, at 1466 (quoting *Cleburne* v. *Cleburne Living Center, Inc.*, 473 U.S. 432, 439 (1985)).

A panel of the Court of Appeals for the Ninth Circuit reversed, emphasizing that "in the two hundred and five years of our existence no constitutional right to aid in killing oneself has ever been asserted and upheld by a court of final jurisdiction." *Compassion in Dying* v. *Washington*, 49 F. 3d 586, 591 (1995). The Ninth Circuit reheard the case en banc, reversed the panel's decision, and affirmed the District Court. *Compassion in Dying* v. *Washington*, 79 F. 3d 790, 798 (1996). Like the District Court, the en banc Court of Appeals emphasized our *Casey* and *Cruzan* decisions. 79 F. 3d, at 813-816. The court also discussed what it described as "historical" and "current societal attitudes" toward suicide and assisted suicide, *id.*, at 806-812, and concluded that "the Constitution encompasses a due process liberty interest in controlling the time and manner of one's death—that there is, in short, a constitutionally recognized 'right to die.'" *Id.*, at 816. After "weighing and then balancing" this interest against Washington's various interests, the court held that the State's assisted suicide ban was unconstitutional "as applied to terminally ill competent adults who wish to hasten their deaths with medication prescribed by their physicians." *Id.*, at 836, 837.[6] The court did not reach the District Court's equal protection holding. *Id.*, at 838.[7] We granted certiorari, 519 U.S. ___ (1996), and now reverse.

I

We begin, as we do in all due process cases, by examining our Nation's history, legal traditions, and practices. See, *e.g.*, *Casey*, 505 U.S., at 849-850; *Cruzan*, 497 U.S., at 269-279; *Moore* v. *East Cleveland*, 431 U.S. 494, 503 (1977) (plurality opinion) (noting importance of "careful 'respect for the teachings of history' "). In almost every State—indeed, in almost every western democracy—it is a crime to assist a suicide.[8] The States' assisted suicide bans are not innovations. Rather, they are longstanding expressions of the States' commitment to the protection and preservation of all human life. *Cruzan,* 497 U.S., at 280 ("The States—indeed, all civilized nations—demonstrate their commitment to life by treating homicide as a serious crime. Moreover, the majority of States in this country have laws imposing criminal penalties on one who assists another to commit suicide"); see *Stanford* v. *Kentucky,* 492 U.S. 361, 373 (1989) ("The primary and most reliable indication of [a national] consensus is . . . the pattern of enacted laws"). Indeed, opposition to and condemnation of suicide—and, therefore, of assisting suicide—are consistent and enduring themes of our philosophical, legal, and cultural heritages. See generally, Marzen, O'Dowd, Crone & Balch, Suicide: A Constitutional Right?, 24 Duquesne L. Rev. 1, 17-56 (1985) (hereinafter Marzen); New York State Task Force on Life and the Law, When Death is Sought: Assisted Suicide and Euthanasia in the Medical Context 77-82 (May 1994) (hereinafter New York Task Force).

More specifically, for over 700 years, the Anglo American common law tradition has punished or otherwise disapproved of both suicide and assisting suicide.[9] *Cruzan,* 497 U.S., at 294-295 (Scalia, J., concurring). In the 13th century, Henry de Bracton, one of the first legal treatise writers, observed that "just as a man may commit felony by slaying another so may he do so by slaying himself." 2 Bracton on Laws and Customs of England 423 (f. 150) (G. Woodbine ed., S. Thorne transl., 1968). The real and personal property of one who killed himself to avoid conviction and punishment for a crime were forfeit to the king; however, thought Bracton, "if a man slays himself in weariness of life or because he is unwilling to endure further bodily pain . . . [only] his movable goods [were] confiscated." *Id.,* at 423-424 (f. 150). Thus, "the principle that suicide of a sane person, for whatever reason, was a punishable felony was . . . introduced into English common law."[10] Centuries later, Sir William Blackstone, whose Commentaries on the Laws of England not only provided a definitive summary of the common law but was also a primary legal authority for 18th and 19th century American lawyers, referred to suicide as "self murder" and "the pretended heroism, but real cowardice, of the Stoic philosophers, who destroyed themselves to avoid those ills which they had not the fortitude to endure. . . . " 4 W. Blackstone, Commentaries *189. Blackstone emphasized that "the law has . . . ranked [suicide] among the highest crimes," *ibid,* although, anticipating later developments, he conceded that the harsh and shameful punishments imposed for suicide "border a little upon severity." *Id.,* at *190.

For the most part, the early American colonies adopted the common law approach. For example, the legislators of the Providence Plantations, which would later become Rhode Island, declared, in 1647, that "self murder is by all agreed to be the most unnatural, and it is by this present Assembly declared, to be that, wherein he that doth it, kills himself out of a premeditated hatred against his own life or other humor: . . . his goods and chattels are the king's custom, but not his debts nor lands; but in case he be an infant, a lunatic, mad or distracted man, he forfeits nothing." The Earliest Acts and Laws of the Colony of Rhode Island and Providence Plantations 1647-1719, p. 19 (J. Cushing ed. 1977). Virginia also required ignominious burial for suicides, and their estates were forfeit to the crown. A. Scott, Criminal Law in Colonial Virginia 108, and n. 93, 198, and n. 15 (1930).

Over time, however, the American colonies abolished these harsh common law penalties. William Penn abandoned the criminal forfeiture sanction in Pennsylvania in 1701, and the other colonies (and later, the other States) eventually followed this example. *Cruzan*, 497 U.S., at 294 (Scalia, J., concurring). Zephaniah Swift, who would later become Chief Justice of Connecticut, wrote in 1796 that "there can be no act more contemptible, than to attempt to punish an offender for a crime, by exercising a mean act of revenge upon lifeless clay, that is insensible of the punishment. There can be no greater cruelty, than the inflicting [of] a punishment, as the forfeiture of goods, which must fall solely on the innocent offspring of the offender. . . . [Suicide] is so abhorrent to the feelings of mankind, and that strong love of life which is implanted in the human heart, that it cannot be so frequently committed, as to become dangerous to society. There can of course be no necessity of any punishment." 2 Z. Swift, A System of the Laws of the State of Connecticut 304 (1796).

This statement makes it clear, however, that the movement away from the common law's harsh sanctions did not represent an acceptance of suicide; rather, as Chief Justice Swift observed, this change reflected the growing consensus that it was unfair to punish the suicide's family for his wrongdoing. *Cruzan, supra*, at 294 (Scalia, J., concurring). Nonetheless, although States moved away from Blackstone's treatment of suicide, courts continued to condemn it as a grave public wrong. See, *e.g., Bigelow* v. *Berkshire Life Ins. Co.*, 93 U.S. 284, 286 (1876) (suicide is "an act of criminal self destruction"); *Von Holden* v. *Chapman*, 87 App. Div. 2d 66, 70-71, 450 N.Y. S. 2d 623, 626-627 (1982); *Blackwood* v. *Jones*, 111 Fla. 528, 532, 149 So. 600, 601 (1933) ("No sophistry is tolerated . . . which seek[s] to justify self-destruction as commendable or even a matter of personal right").

That suicide remained a grievous, though nonfelonious, wrong is confirmed by the fact that colonial and early state legislatures and courts did not retreat from prohibiting assisting suicide. Swift, in his early 19th century treatise on the laws of Connecticut, stated that "[i]f one counsels another to commit suicide, and the other by reason of the advice kills himself, the advisor is guilty of murder as principal." 2 Z. Swift, A Digest of the Laws of the State of Connecticut 270 (1823). This was the well established common law view, see *In re Joseph G.*, 34 Cal. 3d 429, 434-435, 667 P. 2d 1176, 1179 (1983); *Commonwealth* v. *Mink*, 123 Mass. 422, 428 (1877) ("'Now if the murder of one's self is felony, the accessory is equally guilty as if he had aided and abetted in the murder'") (quoting Chief Justice Parker's charge to the jury in *Commonwealth* v. *Bowen*, 13 Mass. 356 (1816)), as was the similar principle that the consent of a homicide victim is "wholly immaterial to the guilt of the person who cause[d] [his death]," 3 J. Stephen, A History of the Criminal Law of England 16 (1883); see 1 F. Wharton, Criminal Law §§451-452 (9th ed. 1885); *Martin* v. *Commonwealth*, 184 Va. 1009, 1018-1019, 37 S. E. 2d 43, 47 (1946) ("'The right to life and to personal security is not only sacred in the estimation of the common law, but it is inalienable'"). And the prohibitions against assisting suicide never contained exceptions for those who were near death. Rather, "the life of those to whom life had become a burden—of those who [were] hopelessly diseased or fatally wounded—nay, even the lives of criminals condemned to death, [were] under the protection of law, equally as the lives of those who [were] in the full tide of life's enjoyment, and anxious to continue to live." *Blackburn* v. *State,* 23 Ohio St. 146, 163 (1872); see *Bowen, supra,* at 360 (prisoner who persuaded another to commit suicide could be tried for murder, even though victim was scheduled shortly to be executed).

The earliest American statute explicitly to outlaw assisting suicide was enacted in New York in 1828, Act of Dec. 10, 1828, ch. 20, §4, 1828 N.Y. Laws 19 (codified at 2 N.Y. Rev. Stat. pt. 4, ch. 1, tit. 2, art. 1, §7, p. 661 (1829)), and many of the new States and Territories followed New York's example. Marzen 73-74. Between 1857 and 1865, a New York commission led by Dudley Field drafted a criminal code that prohibited "aiding" a suicide and, specifically, "furnishing another person with any deadly weapon or poisonous drug, knowing that such person intends to use such weapon or drug in taking his own life." *Id.,* at 76-77. By the time the Fourteenth Amendment was ratified, it was a crime in most States to assist a suicide. See *Cruzan, supra,* at 294-295 (Scalia, J., concurring). The Field Penal Code was adopted in the Dakota Territory in 1877, in New York in 1881, and its language served as a model for several other western States' statutes in the late 19th and early 20th centuries. Marzen 76-77, 205-206, 212-213. California, for example, codified its assisted suicide prohibition in 1874, using language similar to the Field Code's.[11] In this century, the Model Penal Code also prohibited "aiding" suicide, prompting many States to enact or revise their assisted suicide bans.[12] The Code's drafters observed that "the interests in the sanctity of life that are represented by the criminal homicide laws are threatened by one who expresses a willingness to participate in taking the life of another, even though the act may be accomplished with the consent, or at the request, of the suicide victim." American Law Institute, Model Penal Code §210.5, Comment 5, p. 100 (Official Draft and Revised Comments 1980).

Though deeply rooted, the States' assisted suicide bans have in recent years been reexamined and, generally, reaffirmed. Because of advances in medicine and technology, Americans today are increasingly likely to die in institutions, from chronic illnesses. President's Comm'n for the Study of Ethical Problems in Medicine and Biomedical and Behavioral Research, Deciding to Forego Life Sustaining Treatment 16-18 (1983). Public concern and democratic action are therefore sharply focused on how best to protect dignity and independence at the end of life, with the result that there have been many significant changes in state laws and in the attitudes these laws reflect. Many States, for example, now permit "living wills," surrogate health care decision-making, and the withdrawal or refusal of life sustaining medical treatment. See *Vacco* v. *Quill, post,* at 9-11; 79 F. 3d, at 818-820; *People* v. *Kevorkian,* 447 Mich. 436, 478-480, and nn. 53-56, 527 N. W. 2d 714, 731-732, and nn. 53-56 (1994). At the same time, however, voters and legislators continue for the most part to reaffirm their States' prohibitions on assisting suicide.

The Washington statute at issue in this case, Wash. Rev. Code §9A.36.060 (1994), was enacted in 1975 as part of a revision of that State's criminal code. Four years later, Washington passed its Natural Death Act, which specifically stated that the "withholding or withdrawal of life sustaining treatment . . . shall not, for any purpose, constitute a suicide" and that "nothing in this chapter shall be construed to condone, authorize, or approve mercy killing. . . . " Natural Death Act, 1979 Wash. Laws, ch. 112, §§8(1), p. 11 (codified at Wash. Rev. Code §§70.122.070(1), 70.122.100 (1994)). In 1991, Washington voters rejected a ballot initiative which, had it passed, would have permitted a form of physician assisted suicide.[13] Washington then added a provision to the Natural Death Act expressly excluding physician assisted suicide. 1992 Wash. Laws, ch. 98, §10; Wash. Rev. Code §70.122.100 (1994).

California voters rejected an assisted suicide initiative similar to Washington's in 1993. On the other hand, in 1994, voters in Oregon enacted, also through ballot initiative, that State's "Death With Dignity Act," which legalized physician assisted suicide for competent, terminally ill adults.[14] Since the Oregon vote, many proposals to legalize assisted suicide have been and continue to be introduced in the States' legislatures, but none has been enacted.[15] And just last year, Iowa and Rhode Island joined the overwhelming majority of States explicitly prohibiting assisted suicide. See Iowa Code Ann. §§707A.2, 707A.3 (Supp. 1997); R. I. Gen. Laws §§ 11-60-1, 11-60-3 (Supp. 1996). Also, on April 30, 1997, President Clinton signed the Federal Assisted Suicide Funding Restriction Act of 1997, which prohibits the use of federal funds in support of physician assisted suicide. Pub. L. 105-12, 111 Stat. 23 (codified at 42 U.S.C. § 14401 *et seq*).[16]

Thus, the States are currently engaged in serious, thoughtful examinations of physician-assisted suicide and other similar issues. For example, New York State's Task Force on Life and the Law—an ongoing, blue ribbon commission composed of doctors, ethicists, lawyers, religious leaders, and interested laymen—was convened in 1984 and commissioned with "a broad mandate to recommend public policy on issues raised by medical advances." New York Task Force vii. Over the past decade, the Task Force has recommended laws relating to end of life decisions, surrogate pregnancy, and organ donation. *Id.*, at 118-119. After studying physician-assisted suicide, however, the Task Force unanimously concluded that "legalizing assisted suicide and euthanasia would pose profound risks to many individuals who are ill and vulnerable. . . . The potential dangers of this dramatic change in public policy would outweigh any benefit that might be achieved." *Id.*, at 120.

Attitudes toward suicide itself have changed since Bracton, but our laws have consistently condemned, and continue to prohibit, assisting suicide. Despite changes in medical technology and notwithstanding an increased emphasis on the importance of end of life decision-making, we have not retreated from this prohibition. Against this backdrop of history, tradition, and practice, we now turn to respondents' constitutional claim.

II

The Due Process Clause guarantees more than fair process, and the "liberty" it protects includes more than the absence of physical restraint. *Collins* v. *Harker Heights,* 503 U.S. 115, 125 (1992) (Due Process Clause "protects individual liberty against 'certain government actions regardless of the fairness of the procedures used to implement them' ") (quoting *Daniels* v. *Williams*, 474 U.S. 327, 331 (1986)). The Clause also provides heightened protection against government interference with certain fundamental rights and liberty interests. *Reno* v. *Flores*, 507 U.S. 292, 301-302 (1993); *Casey*, 505 U.S., at 851. In a long line of cases, we have held that, in addition to the specific freedoms protected by the Bill of Rights, the "liberty" specially protected by the Due Process Clause includes the rights to marry, *Loving* v. *Virginia*, 388 U.S. 1 (1967); to have children, *Skinner* v. *Oklahoma ex rel. Williamson*, 316 U.S. 535 (1942); to direct the education and upbringing of one's children, *Meyer* v. *Nebraska*, 262 U.S. 390 (1923); *Pierce* v. *Society of Sisters*, 268 U.S. 510 (1925); to marital privacy, *Griswold* v. *Connecticut*, 381 U.S. 479 (1965); to use contraception, *ibid; Eisenstadt* v. *Baird*, 405 U.S. 438 (1972); to bodily integrity, *Rochin* v. *California*, 342 U.S. 165 (1952), and to abortion, *Casey, supra*. We have also assumed, and strongly suggested, that the Due Process Clause protects the traditional right to refuse unwanted lifesaving medical treatment. *Cruzan*, 497 U.S., at 278-279.

But we "have always been reluctant to expand the concept of substantive due process because guideposts for responsible decision-making in this unchartered area are scarce and open ended." *Collins*, 503 U.S., at 125. By extending constitutional protection to an asserted right or liberty interest, we, to a great extent, place the matter outside the arena of public debate and legislative action. We must therefore "exercise the utmost care whenever we are asked to break new ground in this field," *ibid*, lest the liberty protected by the Due Process Clause be subtly transformed into the policy preferences of the members of this Court, *Moore*, 431 U.S., at 502 (plurality opinion).

Our established method of substantive due process analysis has two primary features: First, we have regularly observed that the Due Process Clause specially protects those fundamental rights and liberties which are, objectively, "deeply rooted in this Nation's history and tradition," *id.*, at 503 (plurality opinion); *Snyder* v. *Massachusetts*, 291 U.S. 97, 105 (1934) ("so rooted in the traditions and conscience of our people as to be ranked as fundamental"), and "implicit in the concept of ordered liberty," such that "neither liberty nor justice would exist if they were sacrificed," *Palko* v. *Connecticut*, 302 U.S. 319, 325, 326 (1937). Second, we have required in substantive due process cases a "careful description" of the asserted fundamental liberty interest. *Flores, supra*, at 302; *Collins, supra*, at 125; *Cruzan, supra*, at 277-278. Our Nation's history, legal traditions, and practices thus provide the crucial "guideposts for responsible decision-making," *Collins, supra*, at 125, that direct and restrain our exposition of the Due Process Clause. As we stated recently in *Flores*, the Fourteenth Amendment "forbids the government to infringe . . . 'fundamental' liberty interests *at all*, no matter what process is provided, unless the infringement is narrowly tailored to serve a compelling state interest." 507 U.S., at 302.

Justice Souter, relying on Justice Harlan's dissenting opinion in *Poe* v. *Ullman*, would largely abandon this restrained methodology, and instead ask "whether [Washington's] statute sets up one of those 'arbitrary impositions' or 'purposeless restraints' at odds with the Due Process Clause of the Fourteenth Amendment," *post*, at 1 (quoting *Poe*, 367 U.S. 497, 543 (1961) (Harlan, J., dissenting)).[17] In our view, however, the development of this Court's substantive due process jurisprudence, described briefly above, *supra*, at 15, has been a process whereby the outlines of the "liberty" specially protected by the Fourteenth Amendment—never fully clarified, to be sure, and perhaps not capable of being fully clarified—have at least been carefully refined by concrete examples involving fundamental rights found to be deeply rooted in our legal tradition. This approach tends to rein in the subjective elements that are necessarily present in due process judicial review. In addition, by establishing a threshold requirement—that a challenged state action implicate a fundamental right—before requiring more than a reasonable relation to a legitimate state interest to justify the action, it avoids the need for complex balancing of competing interests in every case.

Turning to the claim at issue here, the Court of Appeals stated that "properly analyzed, the first issue to be resolved is whether there is a liberty interest in determining the time and manner of one's death," 79 F. 3d, at 801, or, in other words, "is there a right to die?," *id.*, at 799. Similarly, respondents assert a "liberty to choose how to die" and a right to "control of one's final days," Brief for Respondents 7, and describe the asserted liberty as "the right to choose a humane, dignified death," *id.*, at 15, and "the liberty to shape death," *id.*, at 18. As noted above, we have a tradition of carefully formulating the interest at stake in substantive due process cases. For example, although *Cruzan* is often described as a "right to die" case, see 79 F. 3d, at 799; *post*, at 9 (Stevens, J., concurring in judgment) (*Cruzan* recognized "the more specific interest in making decisions about how to confront an imminent death"), we were, in fact, more precise: we assumed that the Constitution granted competent persons a "constitutionally protected right to refuse lifesaving hydration and nutrition." *Cruzan*, 497 U.S., at 279; *id.*, at 287 (O'Connor, J., concurring) ("[A] liberty interest in refusing unwanted medical treatment may be inferred from our prior decisions"). The Washington statute at issue in this case prohibits "aiding another person to attempt suicide," Wash. Rev. Code §9A.36.060(1) (1994), and, thus, the question before us is whether the "liberty" specially protected by the Due Process Clause includes a right to commit suicide which itself includes a right to assistance in doing so.[18]

We now inquire whether this asserted right has any place in our Nation's traditions. Here, as discussed above, *supra*, at 4-15, we are confronted with a consistent and almost universal tradition that has long rejected the asserted right, and continues explicitly to reject it today, even for terminally ill, mentally competent adults. To hold for respondents, we would have to reverse centuries of legal doctrine and practice, and strike down the considered policy choice of almost every State. See *Jackman* v. *Rosenbaum Co.*, 260 U.S. 22, 31 (1922) ("If a thing has been practiced for two hundred years by common consent, it will need a strong case for the Fourteenth Amendment to affect it"); *Flores*, 507 U.S., at 303 ("The mere novelty of such a claim is reason enough to doubt that 'substantive due process' sustains it").

Respondents contend, however, that the liberty interest they assert *is* consistent with this Court's substantive due process line of cases, if not with this Nation's history and practice. Pointing to *Casey* and *Cruzan*, respondents read our jurisprudence in this area as reflecting a general tradition of "self sovereignty," Brief of Respondents 12, and as teaching that the "liberty" protected by the Due Process Clause includes "basic and intimate exercises of personal autonomy," *id.*, at 10; see *Casey*, 505 U.S., at 847 ("It is a promise of the Constitution that there is a realm of personal liberty which the government may not enter"). According to respondents, our liberty jurisprudence, and the broad, individualistic principles it reflects, protects the "liberty of competent, terminally ill adults to make end of life decisions free of undue government interference." Brief for Respondents 10. The question presented in this case, however, is whether the protections of the Due Process Clause include a right to commit suicide with another's assistance. With this "careful description" of respondents' claim in mind, we turn to *Casey* and *Cruzan*.

In *Cruzan*, we considered whether Nancy Beth Cruzan, who had been severely injured in an automobile accident and was in a persistive vegetative state, "had a right under the United States Constitution which would require the hospital to withdraw life sustaining treatment" at her parents' request. *Cruzan*, 497 U.S., at 269. We began with the observation that "at common law, even the touching of one person by another without consent and without legal justification was a battery." *Ibid.* We then discussed the related rule that "informed consent is generally required for medical treatment." *Ibid.* After reviewing a long line of relevant state cases, we concluded that "the common law doctrine of informed consent is viewed as generally encompassing the right of a competent individual to refuse medical treatment." *Id.*, at 277. Next, we reviewed our own cases on the subject, and stated that "[t]he principle that a competent person has a constitutionally protected liberty interest in refusing unwanted medical treatment may be inferred from our prior decisions." *Id.*, at 278. Therefore, "for purposes of [that] case, we assume[d] that the United States Constitution would grant a competent person a constitutionally protected right to refuse lifesaving hydration and nutrition." *Id.*, at 279; see *id.*, at 287 (O'Connor, J., concurring). We concluded that, notwithstanding this right, the Constitution permitted Missouri to require clear and convincing evidence of an incompetent patient's wishes concerning the withdrawal of life sustaining treatment. *Id.*, at 280-281.

Respondents contend that in *Cruzan* we "acknowledged that competent, dying persons have the right to direct the removal of life sustaining medical treatment and thus hasten death," Brief for Respondents 23, and that "the constitutional principle behind recognizing the patient's liberty to direct the withdrawal of artificial life support applies at least as strongly to the choice to hasten impending death by consuming lethal medication," *id.*, at 26. Similarly, the Court of Appeals concluded that "*Cruzan*, by recognizing a liberty interest that includes the refusal of artificial provision of life sustaining food and water, necessarily recognized a liberty interest in hastening one's own death." 79 F. 3d, at 816.

The right assumed in *Cruzan*, however, was not simply deduced from abstract concepts of personal autonomy. Given the common law rule that forced medication was a battery, and the long legal tradition protecting the decision to refuse unwanted medical treatment, our assumption was entirely consistent with this Nation's history and constitutional traditions. The decision to commit suicide with the assistance of another may be just as personal and profound as the decision to refuse unwanted medical treatment, but it has never enjoyed similar legal protection. Indeed, the two acts are widely and reasonably regarded as quite distinct. See *Quill* v. *Vacco, post,* at 5-13. In *Cruzan* itself, we recognized that most States outlawed assisted suicide—and even more do today—and we certainly gave no intimation that the right to refuse unwanted medical treatment could be somehow transmuted into a right to assistance in committing suicide. 497 U.S., at 280.

Respondents also rely on *Casey.* There, the Court's opinion concluded that "the essential holding of *Roe* v. *Wade* should be retained and once again reaffirmed." *Casey,* 505 U.S., at 846. We held, first, that a woman has a right, before her fetus is viable, to an abortion "without undue interference from the State"; second, that States may restrict post-viability abortions, so long as exceptions are made to protect a woman's life and health; and third, that the State has legitimate interests throughout a pregnancy in protecting the health of the woman and the life of the unborn child. *Ibid.* In reaching this conclusion, the opinion discussed in some detail this Court's substantive due process tradition of interpreting the Due Process Clause to protect certain fundamental rights and "personal decisions relating to marriage, procreation, contraception, family relationships, child rearing, and education," and noted that many of those rights and liberties "involve the most intimate and personal choices a person may make in a lifetime." *Id.,* at 851.

The Court of Appeals, like the District Court, found *Casey* "'highly instructive'" and "'almost prescriptive'" for determining "'what liberty interest may inhere in a terminally ill person's choice to commit suicide'":

"Like the decision of whether or not to have an abortion, the decision how and when to die is one of 'the most intimate and personal choices a person may make in a lifetime,' a choice 'central to personal dignity and autonomy.'" 79 F. 3d, at 813-814.

Similarly, respondents emphasize the statement in *Casey* that:

"At the heart of liberty is the right to define one's own concept of existence, of meaning, of the universe, and of the mystery of human life. Beliefs about these matters could not define the attributes of personhood were they formed under compulsion of the State." *Casey,* 505 U.S., at 851.

Brief for Respondents 12. By choosing this language, the Court's opinion in *Casey* described, in a general way and in light of our prior cases, those personal activities and decisions that this Court has identified as so deeply rooted in our history and traditions, or so fundamental to our concept of constitutionally ordered liberty, that they are protected by the Fourteenth Amendment.[19] The opinion moved from the recognition that liberty necessarily includes freedom of conscience and belief about ultimate considerations to the observation that "though the abortion decision may originate within the zone of conscience and belief, it is *more than a philosophic exercise.*" *Casey,* 505 U.S., at 852 (emphasis added). That many of the rights and liberties protected by the Due Process Clause sound in personal autonomy does not warrant the sweeping conclusion that any and all important, intimate, and personal decisions are so protected, *San Antonio Independent School Dist.* v. *Rodriguez*, 411 U.S. 1, 33-35 (1973), and *Casey* did not suggest otherwise.

The history of the law's treatment of assisted suicide in this country has been and continues to be one of the rejection of nearly all efforts to permit it. That being the case, our decisions lead us to conclude that the asserted "right" to assistance in committing suicide is not a fundamental liberty interest protected by the Due Process Clause. The Constitution also requires, however, that Washington's assisted suicide ban be rationally related to legitimate government interests. See *Heller* v. *Doe*, 509 U.S. 312, 319-320 (1993); *Flores*, 507 U.S., at 305. This requirement is unquestionably met here. As the court below recognized, 79 F. 3d, at 816-817,[20] Washington's assisted suicide ban implicates a number of state interests.[21] See 49 F. 3d, at 592-593; Brief for State of California et al. as *Amici Curiae* 26-29; Brief for United States as *Amicus Curiae* 16-27.

First, Washington has an "unqualified interest in the preservation of human life." *Cruzan*, 497 U.S., at 282. The State's prohibition on assisted suicide, like all homicide laws, both reflects and advances its commitment to this interest. See *id.*, at 280; Model Penal Code §210.5, Comment 5, at 100 ("The interests in the sanctity of life that are represented by the criminal homicide laws are threatened by one who expresses a willingness to participate in taking the life of another").[22] This interest is symbolic and aspirational as well as practical:

"While suicide is no longer prohibited or penalized, the ban against assisted suicide and euthanasia shores up the notion of limits in human relationships. It reflects the gravity with which we view the decision to take one's own life or the life of another, and our reluctance to encourage or promote these decisions." New York Task Force 131-132.

Respondents admit that "the State has a real interest in preserving the lives of those who can still contribute to society and enjoy life." Brief for Respondents 35, n. 23. The Court of Appeals also recognized Washington's interest in protecting life, but held that the "weight" of this interest depends on the "medical condition and the wishes of the person whose life is at stake." 79 F. 3d, at 817. Washington, however, has rejected this sliding scale approach and, through its assisted suicide ban, insists that all persons' lives, from beginning to end, regardless of physical or mental condition, are under the full protection of the law. See *United States* v. *Rutherford*, 442 U.S. 544, 558 (1979) (". . . Congress could reasonably have determined to protect the terminally ill, no less than other patients, from the vast range of self styled panaceas that inventive minds can devise"). As we have previously affirmed, the States "may properly decline to make judgments about the 'quality' of life that a particular individual may enjoy," *Cruzan*, 497 U.S., at 282. This remains true, as *Cruzan* makes clear, even for those who are near death.

Relatedly, all admit that suicide is a serious public health problem, especially among persons in otherwise vulnerable groups. See Washington State Dept. of Health, Annual Summary of Vital Statistics 1991, pp. 29-30 (Oct. 1992) (suicide is a leading cause of death in Washington of those between the ages of 14 and 54); New York Task Force 10, 23-33 (suicide rate in the general population is about one percent, and suicide is especially prevalent among the young and the elderly). The State has an interest in preventing suicide, and in studying, identifying, and treating its causes. See 79 F. 3d, at 820; *id.*, at 854 (Beezer, J., dissenting) ("The state recognizes suicide as a manifestation of medical and psychological anguish"); Marzen 107-146.

Those who attempt suicide—terminally ill or not—often suffer from depression or other mental disorders. See New York Task Force 13-22, 126-128 (more than 95% of those who commit suicide had a major psychiatric illness at the time of death; among the terminally ill, uncontrolled pain is a "risk factor" because it contributes to depression); Physician Assisted Suicide and Euthanasia in the Netherlands: A Report of Chairman Charles T. Canady to the Subcommittee on the Constitution of the House Committee on the Judiciary, 104th Cong., 2d Sess., 10-11 (Comm. Print 1996); cf. Back, Wallace, Starks, & Pearlman, Physician Assisted Suicide and Euthanasia in Washington State, 275 JAMA 919, 924 (1996) ("Intolerable physical symptoms are not the reason most patients request physician assisted suicide or euthanasia"). Research indicates, however, that many people who request physician-assisted suicide withdraw that request if their depression and pain are treated. H. Hendin, Seduced by Death: Doctors, Patients and the Dutch Cure 24-25 (1997) (suicidal, terminally ill patients "usually respond well to treatment for depressive illness and pain medication and are then grateful to be alive"); New York Task Force 177-178. The New York Task Force, however, expressed its concern that, because depression is difficult to diagnose, physicians and medical professionals often fail to respond adequately to seriously ill patients' needs. *Id.*, at 175. Thus, legal physician assisted suicide could make it more difficult for the State to protect depressed or mentally ill persons, or those who are suffering from untreated pain, from suicidal impulses.

The State also has an interest in protecting the integrity and ethics of the medical profession. In contrast to the Court of Appeals' conclusion that "the integrity of the medical profession would [not] be threatened in any way by [physician assisted suicide]," 79 F. 3d, at 827, the American Medical Association, like many other medical and physicians' groups, has concluded that "physician assisted suicide is fundamentally incompatible with the physician's role as healer." American Medical Association, Code of Ethics §2.211 (1994); see Council on Ethical and Judicial Affairs, Decisions Near the End of Life, 267 JAMA 2229, 2233 (1992) ("The societal risks of involving physicians in medical interventions to cause patients' deaths is too great"); New York Task Force 103-109 (discussing physicians' views). And physician assisted suicide could, it is argued, undermine the trust that is essential to the doctor patient relationship by blurring the time honored line between healing and harming. Assisted Suicide in the United States, Hearing before the Subcommittee on the Constitution of the House Committee on the Judiciary, 104th Cong., 2d Sess., 355-356 (1996) (testimony of Dr. Leon R. Kass) ("The patient's trust in the doctor's whole hearted devotion to his best interests will be hard to sustain").

Next, the State has an interest in protecting vulnerable groups—including the poor, the elderly, and disabled persons—from abuse, neglect, and mistakes. The Court of Appeals dismissed the State's concern that disadvantaged persons might be pressured into physician assisted suicide as "ludicrous on its face." 79 F. 3d, at 825. We have recognized, however, the real risk of subtle coercion

and undue influence in end of life situations. *Cruzan*, 497 U.S., at 281. Similarly, the New York Task Force warned that "legalizing physician assisted suicide would pose profound risks to many individuals who are ill and vulnerable.
. . . The risk of harm is greatest for the many individuals in our society whose autonomy and well being are already compromised by poverty, lack of access to good medical care, advanced age, or membership in a stigmatized social group." New York Task Force 120; see *Compassion in Dying*, 49 F. 3d, at 593 ("An insidious bias against the handicapped—again coupled with a cost saving mentality—makes them especially in need of Washington's statutory protection"). If physician assisted suicide were permitted, many might resort to it to spare their families the substantial financial burden of end of life health care costs.

The State's interest here goes beyond protecting the vulnerable from coercion; it extends to protecting disabled and terminally ill people from prejudice, negative and inaccurate stereotypes, and "societal indifference." 49 F. 3d, at 592. The State's assisted suicide ban reflects and reinforces its policy that the lives of terminally ill, disabled, and elderly people must be no less valued than the lives of the young and healthy, and that a seriously disabled person's suicidal impulses should be interpreted and treated the same way as anyone else's. See New York Task Force 101-102; Physician Assisted Suicide and Euthanasia in the Netherlands: A Report of Chairman Charles T. Canady, at 9, 20 (discussing prejudice toward the disabled and the negative messages euthanasia and assisted suicide send to handicapped patients).

Finally, the State may fear that permitting assisted suicide will start it down the path to voluntary and perhaps even involuntary euthanasia. The Court of Appeals struck down Washington's assisted suicide ban only "as applied to competent, terminally ill adults who wish to hasten their deaths by obtaining medication prescribed by their doctors." 79 F. 3d, at 838. Washington insists, however, that the impact of the court's decision will not and cannot be so limited. Brief for Petitioners 44-47. If suicide is protected as a matter of constitutional right, it is argued, "every man and woman in the United States must enjoy it." *Compassion in Dying*, 49 F. 3d, at 591; see *Kevorkian*, 447 Mich., at 470, n. 41, 527 N. W. 2d, at 727-728, n. 41. The Court of Appeals' decision, and its expansive reasoning, provide ample support for the State's concerns. The court noted, for example, that the "decision of a duly appointed surrogate decision maker is for all legal purposes the decision of the patient himself," 79 F. 3d, at 832, n. 120; that "in some instances, the patient may be unable to self administer the drugs and . . . administration by the physician . . . may be the only way the patient may be able to receive them," *id.*, at 831; and that not only physicians, but also family members and loved ones, will inevitably participate in assisting suicide. *Id.*, at 838, n. 140. Thus, it turns out that what is couched as a limited right to "physician assisted suicide" is likely, in effect, a much broader license, which could prove extremely difficult to police and contain.[23] Washington's ban on assisting suicide prevents such erosion.

This concern is further supported by evidence about the practice of euthanasia in the Netherlands. The Dutch government's own study revealed that in 1990, there were 2,300 cases of voluntary euthanasia (defined as "the deliberate termination of another's life at his request"), 400 cases of assisted suicide, and more than 1,000 cases of euthanasia without an explicit request. In addition to these latter 1,000 cases, the study found an additional 4,941 cases where physicians administered lethal morphine overdoses without the patients' explicit consent. Physician Assisted Suicide and Euthanasia in the Netherlands: A Report of Chairman Charles T. Canady, at 12-13 (citing Dutch study). This study suggests that, despite the existence of various reporting procedures, euthanasia in the Netherlands has not been limited to competent, terminally ill adults who are enduring physical suffering, and that regulation of the practice may not have prevented abuses in cases involving vulnerable persons, including severely disabled neonates and elderly persons suffering from dementia. Id., at 16-21; see generally C. Gomez, Regulating Death: Euthanasia and the Case of the Netherlands (1991); H. Hendin, Seduced By Death: Doctors, Patients, and the Dutch Cure (1997). The New York Task Force, citing the Dutch experience, observed that "assisted suicide and euthanasia are closely linked," New York Task Force 145, and concluded that the "risk of . . . abuse is neither speculative nor distant," id., at 134. Washington, like most other States, reasonably ensures against this risk by banning, rather than regulating, assisting suicide. See United States v. 12 200-ft Reels of Super 8MM Film, 413 U.S. 123, 127 (1973) ("Each step, when taken, appear[s] a reasonable step in relation to that which preceded it, although the aggregate or end result is one that would never have been seriously considered in the first instance").

We need not weigh exactly the relative strengths of these various interests. They are unquestionably important and legitimate, and Washington's ban on assisted suicide is at least reasonably related to their promotion and protection. We therefore hold that Wash. Rev. Code §9A.36.060(1) (1994) does not violate the Fourteenth Amendment, either on its face or "as applied to competent, terminally ill adults who wish to hasten their deaths by obtaining medication prescribed by their doctors." 79 F. 3d, at 838.[24]

* * *

Throughout the Nation, Americans are engaged in an earnest and profound debate about the morality, legality, and practicality of physician assisted suicide. Our holding permits this debate to continue, as it should in a democratic society. The decision of the en banc Court of Appeals is reversed, and the case is remanded for further proceedings consistent with this opinion.

It is so ordered.

NOTES

1. Act of Apr. 28, 1854, §17, 1854 Wash. Laws 78 ("Every person deliberately assisting another in the commission of self murder, shall be deemed guilty of manslaughter"); see also Act of Dec. 2, 1869, §17, 1869 Wash. Laws 201; Act of Nov. 10, 1873, §19, 1873 Wash. Laws 184; Criminal Code, ch. 249, §§135-136, 1909 Wash. Laws, 11th sess., 929.

2. Under Washington's Natural Death Act, "adult persons have the fundamental right to control the decisions relating to the rendering of their own

health care, including the decision to have life sustaining treatment withheld or withdrawn in instances of a terminal condition or permanent unconscious condition." Wash. Rev. Code §70.122.010 (1994). In Washington, "any adult person may execute a directive directing the withholding or withdrawal of life sustaining treatment in a terminal condition or permanent unconscious condition," §70.122.030, and a physician who, in accordance with such a directive, participates in the withholding or withdrawal of life sustaining treatment is immune from civil, criminal, or professional liability. §70.122.051.

3. Glucksberg Declaration, App. 35; Halperin Declaration, *id.*, at 49-50; Preston Declaration, *id.*, at 55-56; Shalit Declaration, *id.*, at 73-74.

4. John Doe, Jane Roe, and James Poe, plaintiffs in the District Court, were then in the terminal phases of serious and painful illnesses. They declared that they were mentally competent and desired assistance in ending their lives. Declaration of Jane Roe, *id.*, at 23-25; Declaration of John Doe, *id.*, at 27-28; Declaration of James Poe, *id.*, at 30-31; *Compassion in Dying*, 850 F. Supp., at 1456-1457.

5. The District Court determined that *Casey's* "undue burden" standard, 505 U.S., at 874 (joint opinion), not the standard from *United States* v. *Salerno*, 481 U.S. 739, 745 (1987) (requiring a showing that "no set of circumstances exists under which the [law] would be valid"), governed the plaintiffs' facial challenge to the assisted suicide ban. 850 F. Supp., at 1462-1464.

6. Although, as Justice Stevens observes, *post*, at 2-3 (opinion concurring in judgment), "[the court's] analysis and eventual holding that the statute was unconstitutional was not limited to a particular set of plaintiffs before it," the court did note that "declaring a statute unconstitutional as applied to members of a group is atypical but not uncommon." 79 F. 3d, at 798, n. 9, and emphasized that it was "not deciding the facial validity of [the Washington statute]," *id.*, at 797-798, and nn. 8-9. It is therefore the court's holding that Washington's physician assisted suicide statute is unconstitutional as applied to the "class of terminally ill, mentally competent patients," *post*, at 14 (Stevens, J., concurring in judgment), that is before us today.

7. The Court of Appeals did note, however, that "the equal protection argument relied on by [the District Court] is not insubstantial," 79 F. 3d., at 838, n. 139, and sharply criticized the opinion in a separate case then pending before the Ninth Circuit, *Lee* v. *Oregon*, 891 F. Supp. 1429 (Ore. 1995) (Oregon's Death With Dignity Act, which permits physician assisted suicide, violates the Equal Protection Clause because it does not provide adequate safeguards against abuse), vacated, *Lee* v. *Oregon*, 107 F. 3d 1382 (CA9 1997) (concluding that plaintiffs lacked Article III standing). *Lee*, of course, is not before us, any more than it was before the Court of Appeals below, and we offer no opinion as to the validity of the *Lee* courts' reasoning. In *Vacco* v. *Quill, post*, however, decided today, we hold that New York's assisted suicide ban does not violate the Equal Protection Clause.

8. See *Compassion in Dying* v. *Washington*, 79 F. 3d 790, 847, and nn. 10-13 (CA9 1996) (Beezer, J., dissenting) ("In total, forty four states, the District of Columbia and two territories prohibit or condemn assisted suicide") (citing

statutes and cases); *Rodriguez* v. *British Columbia (Attorney General)*, 107 D. L. R. (4th) 342, 404 (Can. 1993) ("[A] blanket prohibition on assisted suicide . . . is the norm among western democracies") (discussing assisted suicide provisions in Austria, Spain, Italy, the United Kingdom, the Netherlands, Denmark, Switzerland, and France). Since the Ninth Circuit's decision, Louisiana, Rhode Island, and Iowa have enacted statutory assisted suicide bans. La. Rev. Stat. Ann. §14:32.12 (Supp. 1997); R. I. Gen. Laws §§11-60-1, 11-60-3 (Supp. 1996); Iowa Code Ann. §§707A.2, 707A.3 (Supp. 1997). For a detailed history of the States' statutes, see Marzen, O'Dowd, Crone & Balch, Suicide: A Constitutional Right?, 24 Duquesne L. Rev. 1, 148-242 (1985) (Appendix) (hereinafter Marzen).

9. The common law is thought to have emerged through the expansion of pre-Norman institutions sometime in the 12th century. J. Baker, An Introduction to English Legal History 11 (2d ed. 1979). England adopted the ecclesiastical prohibition on suicide five centuries earlier, in the year 673 at the Council of Hereford, and this prohibition was reaffirmed by King Edgar in 967. See G. Williams, The Sanctity of Life and the Criminal Law 257 (1957).

10. Marzen 59. Other late medieval treatise writers followed and restated Bracton; one observed that "man slaughter" may be "of [one]self; as in case, when people hang themselves or hurt themselves, or otherwise kill themselves of their own felony" or "[o]f others; as by beating, famine, or other punishment; in like cases, all are man slayers." A. Horne, The Mirrour of Justices, ch. 1, §9, pp. 41-42 (W. Robinson ed. 1903). By the mid 16th century, the Court at Common Bench could observe that "[suicide] is an Offence against Nature, against God, and against the King. . . . [T]o destroy one's self is contrary to Nature, and a Thing most horrible." *Hales* v. *Petit*, 1 Plowd. Com. 253, 261, 75 Eng. Rep. 387, 400 (1561-1562).

In 1644, Sir Edward Coke published his Third Institute, a lodestar for later common lawyers. See T. Plucknett, A Concise History of the Common Law 281-284 (5th ed. 1956). Coke regarded suicide as a category of murder, and agreed with Bracton that the goods and chattels—but not, for Coke, the lands—of a sane suicide were forfeit. 3 E. Coke, Institutes *54. William Hawkins, in his 1716 Treatise of the Pleas of the Crown, followed Coke, observing that "our laws have always had . . . an abhorrence of this crime." 1 W. Hawkins, Pleas of the Crown, ch. 27, §4, p. 164 (T. Leach ed. 1795).

11. In 1850, the California legislature adopted the English common law, under which assisting suicide was, of course, a crime. Act of Apr. 13, 1850, ch. 95, 1850 Cal. Stats. 219. The provision adopted in 1874 provided that "every person who deliberately aids or advises, or encourages another to commit suicide, is guilty of a felony." Act of Mar. 30, 1874, ch. 614, §13, 400, 255 (codified at Cal. Penal Code §400 (T. Hittel ed. 1876)).

12. "A person who purposely aids or solicits another to commit suicide is guilty of a felony in the second degree if his conduct causes such suicide or an attempted suicide, and otherwise of a misdemeanor." American Law Institute, Model Penal Code §210.5(2) (Official Draft and Revised Comments 1980).

13. Initiative 119 would have amended Washington's Natural Death Act, Wash. Rev. Code §70.122.010 *et seq.* (1994), to permit "aid in dying", defined as "aid in the form of a medical service provided in person by a physician that will end the life of a conscious and mentally competent qualified patient in a dignified, painless and humane manner, when requested voluntarily by the patient through a written directive in accordance with this chapter at the time the medical service is to be provided." App. H to Pet. for Cert. 3-4.

14. Ore. Rev. Stat. §§127.800 *et seq.* (1996); *Lee* v. *Oregon*, 891 F. Supp. 1429 (Ore. 1995) (Oregon Act does not provide sufficient safeguards for terminally ill persons and therefore violates the Equal Protection Clause), vacated, *Lee* v. *Oregon*, 107 F. 3d 1382 (CA9 1997).

15. See, *e.g.*, Alaska H. B. 371 (1996); Ariz. S. B. 1007 (1996); Cal. A. B. 1080, A. B. 1310 (1995); Colo. H. B. 1185 (1996); Colo. H. B. 1308 (1995); Conn. H. B. 6298 (1995); Ill. H. B. 691, S. B. 948 (1997); Me. H. P. 663 (1997); Me. H. P. 552 (1995); Md. H. B. 474 (1996); Md. H. B. 933 (1995); Mass. H. B. 3173 (1995); Mich. H. B. 6205 (1996); Mich. S. B. 556 (1996); Mich. H. B. 4134 (1995); Miss. H. B. 1023 (1996); N. H. H. B. 339 (1995); N. M. S. B. 446 (1995); N.Y. S. B. 5024 (1995); N.Y. A. B. 6333 (1995); Neb. L. B. 406 (1997); Neb. L. B. 1259 (1996); R. I. S. 2985 (1996); Vt. H. B. 109 (1997); Vt. H. B. 335 (1995); Wash. S. B. 5596 (1995); Wis. A. B. 174, S. B. 90 (1995); Senate of Canada, Of Life and Death, Report of the Special Senate Committee on Euthanasia and Assisted Suicide

A—156 (June 1995) (describing unsuccessful proposals, between 1991-1994, to legalize assisted suicide).

16. Other countries are embroiled in similar debates: The Supreme Court of Canada recently rejected a claim that the Canadian Charter of Rights and Freedoms establishes a fundamental right to assisted suicide, *Rodriguez* v. *British Columbia (Attorney General)*, 107 D. L. R. (4th) 342 (1993); the British House of Lords Select Committee on Medical Ethics refused to recommend any change in Great Britain's assisted suicide prohibition, House of Lords, Session 1993-94 Report of the Select Committee on Medical Ethics, 12 Issues in Law & Med. 193, 202 (1996) ("We identify no circumstances in which assisted suicide should be permitted"); New Zealand's Parliament rejected a proposed "Death With Dignity Bill" that would have legalized physician assisted suicide in August 1995, Graeme, MPs Throw out Euthanasia Bill, The Dominion (Wellington), Aug. 17, 1995, p. 1; and the Northern Territory of Australia legalized assisted suicide and voluntary euthanasia in 1995. See Shenon, Australian Doctors Get Right to Assist Suicide, N.Y. Times, July 28, 1995, p. A8. As of February 1997, three persons had ended their lives with physician assistance in the Northern Territory. Mydans, Assisted Suicide: Australia Faces a Grim Reality, N.Y. Times, Febr. 2, 1997, p. A3. On March 24, 1997, however, the Australian Senate voted to overturn the Northern Territory's law. Thornhill, Australia Repeals Euthanasia Law, Washington Post, March 25, 1997, p. A14; see Euthanasia Laws Act 1997, No. 17, 1997 (Austl.). On the other hand, on May 20, 1997, Colombia's Constitutional Court legalized voluntary euthanasia for terminally ill people. Sentencia No. C 239/97 (Corte Constitucional, Mayo 20,

1997); see Colombia's Top Court Legalizes Euthanasia, Orlando Sentinel, May 22, 1997, p. A18.

17. In Justice Souter's opinion, Justice Harlan's *Poe* dissent supplies the "modern justification" for substantive due process review. *Post*, at 5, and n. 2 (Souter, J., concurring in judgment). But although Justice Harlan's opinion has often been cited in due process cases, we have never abandoned our fundamental rights based analytical method. Just four Terms ago, six of the Justices now sitting joined the Court's opinion in *Reno* v. *Flores*, 507 U.S. 292, 301-305 (1993); *Poe* was not even cited. And in *Cruzan*, neither the Court's nor the concurring opinions relied on *Poe*; rather, we concluded that the right to refuse unwanted medical treatment was so rooted in our history, tradition, and practice as to require special protection under the Fourteenth Amendment. *Cruzan* v. *Director, Mo. Dept. of Health*, 497 U.S. 261, 278-279 (1990); *id.*, at 287-288 (O'Connor, J., concurring). True, the Court relied on Justice Harlan's dissent in *Casey*, 505 U.S., at 848-850, but, as *Flores* demonstrates, we did not in so doing jettison our established approach. Indeed, to read such a radical move into the Court's opinion in *Casey* would seem to fly in the face of that opinion's emphasis on *stare decisis*. 505 U.S., at 854-869.

18. See, *e.g.*, *Quill* v. *Vacco*, 80 F. 3d 716, 724 (CA2 1996) ("right to assisted suicide finds no cognizable basis in the Constitution's language or design"); *Compassion in Dying* v. *Washington*, 49 F. 3d 586, 591 (CA9 1995) (referring to alleged "right to suicide," "right to assistance in suicide," and "right to aid in killing oneself"); *People* v. *Kevorkian*, 447 Mich. 436, 476, n. 47, 527 N. W. 2d 714, 730, n. 47 (1994) ("[T]he question that we must decide is whether the [C]onstitution encompasses a right to commit suicide and, if so, whether it includes a right to assistance").

19. See *Moore* v. *East Cleveland*, 431 U.S. 494, 503 (1977) ("[T]he Constitution protects the sanctity of the family *precisely because* the institution of the family is deeply rooted in this Nation's history and tradition") (emphasis added); *Griswold* v. *Connecticut*, 381 U.S. 479, 485-486 (1965) (intrusions into the "sacred precincts of marital bedrooms" offend rights "older than the Bill of Rights"); *id.*, at 495-496 (Goldberg, J., concurring) (the law in question "disrupted the traditional relation of the family—a relation as old and as fundamental as our entire civilization"); *Loving* v. *Virginia*, 388 U.S. 1, 12 (1967) ("The freedom to marry has long been recognized as one of the vital personal rights essential to the orderly pursuit of happiness"); *Turner* v. *Safley*, 482 U.S. 78, 95 (1987) ("[T]he decision to marry is a fundamental right"); *Roe* v. *Wade*, 410 U.S. 113, 140 (1973) (stating that at the Founding and throughout the 19th century, "a woman enjoyed a substantially broader right to terminate a pregnancy"); *Skinner* v. *Oklahoma ex rel. Williamson*, 316 U.S. 535, 541 (1942) ("Marriage and procreation are fundamental"); *Pierce* v. *Society of Sisters*, 268 U.S. 510, 535 (1925); *Meyer* v. *Nebraska*, 262 U.S. 390, 399 (1923) (liberty includes "those privileges long recognized at common law as essential to the orderly pursuit of happiness by free men").

20. The court identified and discussed six state interests: (1) preserving life; (2) preventing suicide; (3) avoiding the involvement of third parties and use

of arbitrary, unfair, or undue influence; (4) protecting family members and loved ones; (5) protecting the integrity of the medical profession; and (6) avoiding future movement toward euthanasia and other abuses. 79 F. 3d, at 816-832.

21. Respondents also admit the existence of these interests, Brief for Respondents 28-39, but contend that Washington could better promote and protect them through regulation, rather than prohibition, of physician assisted suicide. Our inquiry, however, is limited to the question whether the State's prohibition is rationally related to legitimate state interests.

22. The States express this commitment by other means as well:
"Nearly all states expressly disapprove of suicide and assisted suicide either in statutes dealing with durable powers of attorney in health care situations, or in 'living will' statutes. In addition, all states provide for the involuntary commitment of persons who may harm themselves as the result of mental illness, and a number of states allow the use of nondeadly force to thwart suicide attempts." *People* v. *Kevorkian*, 447 Mich., at 478-479, and nn. 53-56, 527 N. W. 2d, at 731-732, and nn. 53-56.

23. Justice Souter concludes that "[t]he case for the slippery slope is fairly made out here, not because recognizing one due process right would leave a court with no principled basis to avoid recognizing another, but because there is a plausible case that the right claimed would not be readily containable by reference to facts about the mind that are matters of difficult judgment, or by gatekeepers who are subject to temptation, noble or not." *Post*, at 36-37 (opinion concurring in judgment). We agree that the case for a slippery slope has been made out, but—bearing in mind Justice Cardozo's observation of "the tendency of a principle to expand itself to the limit of its logic," The Nature of the Judicial Process 51 (1932)—we also recognize the reasonableness of the widely expressed skepticism about the lack of a principled basis for confining the right. See Brief for United States as *Amicus Curiae* 26 ("Once a legislature abandons a categorical prohibition against physician assisted suicide, there is no obvious stopping point"); Brief for Not Dead Yet et al. as *Amici Curiae* 21-29; Brief for Bioethics Professors as *Amici Curiae* 23-26; Report of the Council on Ethical and Judicial Affairs, App. 133, 140 ("If assisted suicide is permitted, then there is a strong argument for allowing euthanasia"); New York Task Force 132; Kamisar, The "Right to Die": On Drawing (and Erasing) Lines, 35 Duquesne L. Rev. 481 (1996); Kamisar, Against Assisted Suicide— Even in a Very Limited Form, 72 U. Det. Mercy L. Rev. 735 (1995).

24. Justice Stevens states that "the Court does conceive of respondents' claim as a facial challenge—addressing not the application of the statute to a particular set of plaintiffs before it, but the constitutionality of the statute's categorical prohibition. . . . " *Post*, at 4 (opinion concurring in judgment). We emphasize that we today reject the Court of Appeals' specific holding that the statute is unconstitutional "as applied" to a particular class. See n. 6, *supra.* Justice Stevens agrees with this holding, see *post*, at 14, but would not "foreclose the possibility that an individual plaintiff seeking to hasten her death, or a doctor whose assistance was sought, could prevail in a more particularized chal-

lenge," *ibid.* Our opinion does not absolutely foreclose such a claim. However, given our holding that the Due Process Clause of the Fourteenth Amendment does not provide heightened protection to the asserted liberty interest in ending one's life with a physician's assistance, such a claim would have to be quite different from the ones advanced by respondents here.

Supreme Court of the United States

WASHINGTON ET AL., PETITIONERS 96-110 *v.* HAROLD
GLUCKSBERG ET AL.
ON WRIT OF CERTIORARI TO THE UNITED STATES COURT OF APPEALS
FOR THE NINTH CIRCUIT
DENNIS C. VACCO, ATTORNEY GENERAL OF NEW YORK, ET AL.,
PETITIONERS 95-1858 *v.* TIMOTHY E. QUILL ET AL.
ON WRIT OF CERTIORARI TO THE UNITED STATES COURT OF APPEALS
FOR THE SECOND CIRCUIT
[JUNE 26, 1997]

Justice O'Connor, concurring.*

Death will be different for each of us. For many, the last days will be spent in physical pain and perhaps the despair that accompanies physical deterioration and a loss of control of basic bodily and mental functions. Some will seek medication to alleviate that pain and other symptoms.

The Court frames the issue in this case as whether the Due Process Clause of the Constitution protects a "right to commit suicide which itself includes a right to assistance in doing so," *ante,* at 18, and concludes that our Nation's history, legal traditions, and practices do not support the existence of such a right. I join the Court's opinions because I agree that there is no generalized right to "commit suicide." But respondents urge us to address the narrower question whether a mentally competent person who is experiencing great suffering has a constitutionally cognizable interest in controlling the circumstances of his or her imminent death. I see no need to reach that question in the context of the facial challenges to the New York and Washington laws at issue here. See *ante,* at 18 ("The Washington statute at issue in this case prohibits 'aiding another person to attempt suicide,' . . . and, thus, the question before us is whether the 'liberty' specially protected by the Due Process Clause includes a right to commit suicide which itself includes a right to assistance in doing so"). The parties and *amici* agree that in these States a patient who is suffering from a terminal illness and who is experiencing great pain has no legal barriers to obtaining medication, from qualified physicians, to alleviate that suffering, even to the point of causing unconsciousness and hastening death. See Wash. Rev. Code §70.122.010 (1994); Brief for Petitioners in No. 95-1858, p. 15, n. 9; Brief for Respondents in No. 95-1858, p. 15. In this light, even assuming that we would recognize such an interest, I agree that the State's interests in protecting those who are not truly competent or facing imminent death, or those whose decisions to hasten death would not truly be voluntary, are sufficiently weighty to justify a prohibition against physician assisted suicide. *Ante,* at 27-30; *post,* at 11 (Stevens, J., concurring in judgments); *post,* at 33-39 (Souter, J., concurring in judgment).

Every one of us at some point may be affected by our own or a family member's terminal illness. There is no reason to think the democratic process will not strike the proper balance between the interests of terminally ill, mentally competent individuals who would seek to end their suffering and the State's interests in protecting those who might seek to end life mistakenly or under pressure. As the Court recognizes, States are presently undertaking extensive and serious evaluation of physician-assisted suicide and other related issues. *Ante,* at 11, 12-13; see *post,* at 36-39 (Souter, J., concurring in judgment). In such circumstances, "the . . . challenging task of crafting appropriate procedures for safeguarding . . . liberty interests is entrusted to the 'laboratory' of the States . . . in the first instance." *Cruzan* v. *Director, Mo. Dept. of Health,* 497 U.S. 261, 292 (1990) (O'Connor, J., concurring) (citing *New State Ice Co.* v. *Liebmann,* 285 U.S. 262, 311 (1932)).

In sum, there is no need to address the question whether suffering patients have a constitutionally cognizable interest in obtaining relief from the suffering that they may experience in the last days of their lives. There is no dispute that dying patients in Washington and New York can obtain palliative care, even when doing so would hasten their deaths. The difficulty in defining terminal illness and the risk that a dying patient's request for assistance in ending his or her life might not be truly voluntary justifies the prohibitions on assisted suicide we uphold here.

NOTES

* Justice Ginsburg concurs in the Court's judgments substantially for the reasons stated in this opinion. Justice Breyer joins this opinion except insofar as it joins the opinions of the Court.

Supreme Court of the United States

WASHINGTON ET AL., PETITIONERS 96-110 *v.* HAROLD
GLUCKSBERG ET AL.
ON WRIT OF CERTIORARI TO THE UNITED STATES COURT OF APPEALS
FOR THE NINTH CIRCUIT

DENNIS C. VACCO, ATTORNEY GENERAL OF NEW YORK, ET AL.,
PETITIONERS 95-1858 *v.* TIMOTHY E. QUILL ET AL.

ON WRIT OF CERTIORARI TO THE UNITED STATES COURT OF APPEALS
FOR THE SECOND CIRCUIT

[JUNE 26, 1997]

Justice Stevens, concurring in the judgments.

The Court ends its opinion with the important observation that our holding today is fully consistent with a continuation of the vigorous debate about the "morality, legality, and practicality of physician assisted suicide" in a democratic society. *Ante,* at 32. I write separately to make it clear that there is also room for further debate about the limits that the Constitution places on the power of the States to punish the practice.

The morality, legality, and practicality of capital punishment have been the subject of debate for many years. In 1976, this Court upheld the constitutionality of the practice in cases coming to us from Georgia,[1] Florida,[2] and Texas.[3] In those cases we concluded that a State does have the power to place a lesser value on some lives than on others; there is no absolute requirement that a State treat all human life as having an equal right to preservation. Because the state legislatures had sufficiently narrowed the category of lives that the State could terminate, and had enacted special procedures to ensure that the defendant belonged in that limited category, we concluded that the statutes were not unconstitutional on their face. In later cases coming to us from each of those States, however, we found that some applications of the statutes were unconstitutional.[4]

Today, the Court decides that Washington's statute prohibiting assisted suicide is not invalid "on its face," that is to say, in all or most cases in which it might be applied.[5] That holding, however, does not foreclose the possibility that some applications of the statute might well be invalid.

As originally filed, this case presented a challenge to the Washington statute on its face and as it applied to three terminally ill, mentally competent patients and to four physicians who treat terminally ill patients. After the District Court issued its opinion holding that the statute placed an undue burden on the right to commit physician assisted suicide, see *Compassion in Dying* v. *Washington,* 850 F. Supp. 1454, 1462, 1465 (WD Wash. 1994), the three patients died. Although the Court of Appeals considered the constitutionality of the statute-as applied to the prescription of life ending medication for use by terminally ill, competent adult patients who wish to hasten their deaths," *Compassion in Dying* v. *Washington,* 79 F. 3d 790, 798 (CA9 1996), the court did not have before it any individual plaintiff seeking to hasten her death or any doctor who was threatened with prosecution for assisting in the suicide of a particular patient; its analysis and eventual holding that the statute was unconstitutional was not limited to a particular set of plaintiffs before it.

The appropriate standard to be applied in cases making facial challenges to state statutes has been the subject of debate within this Court. See *Janklow v. Planned Parenthood, Sioux Falls Clinic,* 517 U.S. _____ (1996). Upholding the validity of the federal Bail Reform Act of 1984, the Court stated in *United States v. Salerno,* 481 U.S. 739 (1987), that a "facial challenge to a legislative Act is, of course, the most difficult challenge to mount successfully, since the challenger must establish that no set of circumstances exists under which the Act would be valid." *Id.,* at 745.[6] I do not believe the Court has ever actually applied such a strict standard,[7] even in *Salerno* itself, and the Court does not appear to apply *Salerno* here. Nevertheless, the Court does conceive of respondents' claim as a facial challenge—addressing not the application of the statute to a particular set of plaintiffs before it, but the constitutionality of the statute's categorical prohibition against "aiding another person to attempt suicide." *Ante,* at 18 (internal quotation marks omitted) (citing Wash. Rev. Code §9A.36.060(1) (1994)). Accordingly, the Court requires the plaintiffs to show that the interest in liberty protected by the Fourteenth Amendment "includes a right to commit suicide which itself includes a right to assistance in doing so." *Ante,* at 18.

History and tradition provide ample support for refusing to recognize an open ended constitutional right to commit suicide. Much more than the State's paternalistic interest in protecting the individual from the irrevocable consequences of an ill-advised decision motivated by temporary concerns is at stake. There is truth in John Donne's observation that "No man is an island."[8] The State has an interest in preserving and fostering the benefits that every human being may provide to the community—a community that thrives on the exchange of ideas, expressions of affection, shared memories and humorous incidents as well as on the material contributions that its members create and support. The value to others of a person's life is far too precious to allow the individual to claim a constitutional entitlement to complete autonomy in making a decision to end that life. Thus, I fully agree with the Court that the "liberty" protected by the Due Process Clause does not include a categorical "right to commit suicide which itself includes a right to assistance in doing so." *Ante,* at 18.

But just as our conclusion that capital punishment is not always unconstitutional did not preclude later decisions holding that it is sometimes impermissibly cruel, so is it equally clear that a decision upholding a general statutory prohibition of assisted suicide does not mean that every possible application of the statute would be valid. A State, like Washington, that has authorized the death penalty and thereby has concluded that the sanctity of human life does not require that it always be preserved, must acknowledge that there are situations in which an interest in hastening death is legitimate. Indeed, not only is that interest sometimes legitimate, I am also convinced that there are times when it is entitled to constitutional protection.

In *Cruzan v. Director, Mo. Dept. of Health,* 497 U.S. 261 (1990), the Court assumed that the interest in liberty protected by the Fourteenth Amendment encompassed the right of a terminally ill patient to direct the withdrawal of life sustaining treatment. As the Court correctly observes today, that assumption "was not simply deduced from abstract concepts of personal autonomy." *Ante*, at 21. Instead, it was supported by the common law tradition protecting the individual's general right to refuse unwanted medical treatment. *Ibid.* We have recognized, however, that this common law right to refuse treatment is neither absolute nor always sufficiently weighty to overcome valid countervailing state interests. As Justice Brennan pointed out in his *Cruzan* dissent, we have upheld legislation imposing punishment on persons refusing to be vaccinated, 497 U.S., at 312, n. 12, citing *Jacobson* v. *Massachusetts,* 197 U.S. 11, 26-27 (1905), and as Justice Scalia pointed out in his concurrence, the State ordinarily has the right to interfere with an attempt to commit suicide by, for example, forcibly placing a bandage on a self inflicted wound to stop the flow of blood. 497 U.S., at 298. In most cases, the individual's constitutionally protected interest in his or her own physical autonomy, including the right to refuse unwanted medical treatment, will give way to the State's interest in preserving human life.

Cruzan, however, was not the normal case. Given the irreversible nature of her illness and the progressive character of her suffering,[9] Nancy Cruzan's interest in refusing medical care was incidental to her more basic interest in controlling the manner and timing of her death. In finding that her best interests would be served by cutting off the nourishment that kept her alive, the trial court did more than simply vindicate Cruzan's interest in refusing medical treatment; the court, in essence, authorized affirmative conduct that would hasten her death. When this Court reviewed the case and upheld Missouri's requirement that there be clear and convincing evidence establishing Nancy Cruzan's intent to have life sustaining nourishment withdrawn, it made two important assumptions: (1) that there was a "liberty interest" in refusing unwanted treatment protected by the Due Process Clause; and (2) that this liberty interest did not "end the inquiry" because it might be outweighed by relevant state interests. *Id.,* at 279. I agree with both of those assumptions, but I insist that the source of Nancy Cruzan's right to refuse treatment was not just a common law rule. Rather, this right is an aspect of a far broader and more basic concept of freedom that is even older than the common law.[10] This freedom embraces, not merely a person's right to refuse a particular kind of unwanted treatment, but also her interest in dignity, and in determining the character of the memories that will survive long after her death.[11] In recognizing that the State's interests did not outweigh Nancy Cruzan's liberty interest in refusing medical treatment, *Cruzan* rested not simply on the common law right to refuse medical treatment, but—at least implicitly—on the even more fundamental right to make this "deeply personal decision," 497 U.S., at 289 (O'Connor, J., concurring).

Thus, the common law right to protection from battery, which included the right to refuse medical treatment in most circumstances, did not mark "the outer limits of the substantive sphere of liberty" that supported the Cruzan family's decision to hasten Nancy's death. *Planned Parenthood of Southeastern Pa.* v. *Casey,* 505 U.S. 833, 848 (1992). Those limits have never been precisely defined. They are generally identified by the importance and character of the decision confronted by the individual, *Whalen* v. *Roe,* 429 U.S. 589, 599-600, n. 26 (1977). Whatever the outer limits of the concept may be, it definitely includes protection for matters "central to personal dignity and autonomy." *Casey,* 505 U.S., at 851. It includes, "the individual's right to make certain unusually important decisions that will affect his own, or his family's, destiny. The Court has referred to such decisions as implicating 'basic values,' as being 'fundamental,' and as being dignified by history and tradition. The character of the Court's language in these cases brings to mind the origins of the American heritage of freedom—the abiding interest in individual liberty that makes certain state intrusions on the citizen's right to decide how he will live his own life intolerable." *Fitzgerald* v. *Porter Memorial Hospital,* 523 F. 2d 716, 719-720 (CA7 1975) (footnotes omitted), cert. denied, 425 U.S. 916 (1976).

The *Cruzan* case demonstrated that some state intrusions on the right to decide how death will be encountered are also intolerable. The now deceased plaintiffs in this action may in fact have had a liberty interest even stronger than Nancy Cruzan's because, not only were they terminally ill, they were suffering constant and severe pain. Avoiding intolerable pain and the indignity of living one's final days incapacitated and in agony is certainly "at the heart of [the] liberty . . . to define one's own concept of existence, of meaning, of the universe, and of the mystery of human life." *Casey,* 505 U.S., at 851.

While I agree with the Court that *Cruzan* does not decide the issue presented by these cases, *Cruzan* did give recognition, not just to vague, unbridled notions of autonomy, but to the more specific interest in making decisions about how to confront an imminent death. Although there is no absolute right to physician assisted suicide, *Cruzan* makes it clear that some individuals who no longer have the option of deciding whether to live or to die because they are already on the threshold of death have a constitutionally protected interest that may outweigh the State's interest in preserving life at all costs. The liberty interest at stake in a case like this differs from, and is stronger than, both the common law right to refuse medical treatment and the unbridled interest in deciding whether to live or die. It is an interest in deciding how, rather than whether, a critical threshold shall be crossed.

The state interests supporting a general rule banning the practice of physician assisted suicide do not have the same force in all cases. First and foremost of these interests is the " 'unqualified interest in the preservation of human life,' " *ante,* at 24, (quoting *Cruzan,* 497 U.S., at 282,) which is equated with " 'the sanctity of life,' " *ante,* at 25, (quoting the American Law Institute, Model Penal Code §210.5, Comment 5, p. 100 (Official Draft and Revised Comments 1980)). That interest not only justifies—it commands—maximum protection of every individual's interest in remaining alive, which in turn commands the same protection for decisions about whether to commence or to terminate life support systems or to administer pain medication that may hasten death. Properly viewed, however, this interest is not a collective interest that should always outweigh the interests of a person who because of pain, incapacity, or sedation finds her life intolerable, but rather, an aspect of individual freedom.

Many terminally ill people find their lives meaningful even if filled with pain or dependence on others. Some find value in living through suffering; some have an abiding desire to witness particular events in their families' lives; many believe it a sin to hasten death. Individuals of different religious faiths make different judgments and choices about whether to live on under such circumstances. There are those who will want to continue aggressive treatment; those who would prefer terminal sedation; and those who will seek withdrawal from life support systems and death by gradual starvation and dehydration. Although as a general matter the State's interest in the contributions each person may make to society outweighs the person's interest in ending her life, this interest does not have the same force for a terminally ill patient faced not with the choice of whether to live, only of how to die. Allowing the individual, rather than the State, to make judgments "'about the "quality" of life that a particular individual may enjoy.'" *ante,* at 25 (quoting *Cruzan,* 497 U.S., at 282), does not mean that the lives of terminally ill, disabled people have less value than the lives of those who are healthy, see *ante,* at 28. Rather, it gives proper recognition to the individual's interest in choosing a final chapter that accords with her life story, rather than one that demeans her values and poisons memories of her. See Brief for Bioethicists as *Amici Curiae* 11; see also R. Dworkin, Life's Dominion 213 (1993) ("Whether it is in someone's best interests that his life end in one way rather than another depends on so much else that is special about him—about the shape and character of his life and his own sense of his integrity and critical interests—that no uniform collective decision can possibly hope to serve everyone even decently").

Similarly, the State's legitimate interests in preventing suicide, protecting the vulnerable from coercion and abuse, and preventing euthanasia are less significant in this context. I agree that the State has a compelling interest in preventing persons from committing suicide because of depression, or coercion by third parties. But the State's legitimate interest in preventing abuse does not apply to an individual who is not victimized by abuse, who is not suffering from depression, and who makes a rational and voluntary decision to seek assistance in dying. Although, as the New York Task Force report discusses, diagnosing depression and other mental illness is not always easy, mental health workers and other professionals expert in working with dying patients can help patients cope with depression and pain, and help patients assess their options. See Brief for Washington State Psychological Association et al. as *Amici Curiae* 8-10.

Relatedly, the State and *amici* express the concern that patients whose physical pain is inadequately treated will be more likely to request assisted suicide. Encouraging the development and ensuring the availability of adequate pain treatment is of utmost importance; palliative care, however, cannot alleviate all pain and suffering. See Orentlicher, Legalization of Physician Assisted Suicide: A Very Modest Revolution, 38 Boston College L. Rev. (Galley, p. 8) (1997) ("Greater use of palliative care would reduce the demand for assisted suicide, but it will not eliminate [it]"); see also Brief for Coalition of Hospice Professionals as *Amici Curiae* 8 (citing studies showing that "as death becomes more imminent, pain and suffering become progressively more difficult to treat"). An individual adequately informed of the care alternatives thus might make a rational choice for assisted suicide. For such an individual, the State's interest in preventing potential abuse and mistake is only minimally implicated.

The final major interest asserted by the State is its interest in preserving the traditional integrity of the medical profession. The fear is that a rule permitting physicians to assist in suicide is inconsistent with the perception that they serve their patients solely as healers. But for some patients, it would be a physician's refusal to dispense medication to ease their suffering and make their death tolerable and dignified that would be inconsistent with the healing role See Block & Billings, Patient Request to Hasten Death, 154 Archives Internal Med. 2039, 2045 (1994) (A doctor's refusal to hasten death "may be experienced by the [dying] patient as an abandonment, a rejection, or an expression of inappropriate paternalistic authority"). For doctors who have long standing relationships with their patients, who have given their patients advice on alternative treatments, who are attentive to their patient's individualized needs, and who are knowledgeable about pain symptom management and palliative care options, see Quill, Death and Dignity, A Case of Individualized Decision-Making, 324 New England J. of Med. 691-694 (1991), heeding a patient's desire to assist in her suicide would not serve to harm the physician patient relationship. Furthermore, because physicians are already involved in making decisions that hasten the death of terminally ill patients—through termination of life support, withholding of medical treatment, and terminal sedation—there is in fact significant tension between the traditional view of the physician's role and the actual practice in a growing number of cases.[12]

As the New York State Task Force on Life and the Law recognized, a State's prohibition of assisted suicide is justified by the fact that the "'ideal'" case in which "patients would be screened for depression and offered treatment, effective pain medication would be available, and all patients would have a supportive committed family and doctor" is not the usual case. New York State Task Force on Life and the Law, When Death Is Sought: Assisted Suicide and Euthanasia in the Medical Context 120 (May 1994). Although, as the Court concludes today, these *potential* harms are sufficient to support the State's general public policy against assisted suicide, they will not always outweigh the individual liberty interest of a particular patient. Unlike the Court of Appeals, I would not say as a categorical matter that these state interests are invalid as to the entire class of terminally ill, mentally competent patients. I do not, however, foreclose the possibility that an individual plaintiff seeking to hasten her death, or a doctor whose assistance was sought, could prevail in a more particularized challenge. Future cases will determine whether such a challenge may succeed.

In New York, a doctor must respect a competent person's decision to refuse or to discontinue medical treatment even though death will thereby ensue, but the same doctor would be guilty of a felony if she provided her patient assistance in committing suicide.[13] Today we hold that the Equal Protection Clause is not violated by the resulting disparate treatment of two classes of terminally ill people who may have the same interest in hastening death. I agree that the distinction between permitting death to ensue from an underlying fatal disease and causing it to occur by the administration of medication or other means provides a constitutionally sufficient basis for the State's classification.[14] Unlike the Court, however, see *Vacco, ante,* at 6-7, I am not persuaded that in all cases there will in fact be a significant difference between the intent of the physicians, the patients or the families in the two situations.

There may be little distinction between the intent of a terminally ill patient who decides to remove her life support and one who seeks the assistance of a doctor in ending her life; in both situations, the patient is seeking to hasten a certain, impending death. The doctor's intent might also be the same in prescribing lethal medication as it is in terminating life support. A doctor who fails to administer medical treatment to one who is dying from a disease could be doing so with an intent to harm or kill that patient. Conversely, a doctor who prescribes lethal medication does not necessarily intend the patient's death—rather that doctor may seek simply to ease the patient's suffering and to comply with her wishes. The illusory character of any differences in intent or causation is confirmed by the fact that the American Medical Association unequivocally endorses the practice of terminal sedation—the administration of sufficient dosages of pain killing medication to terminally ill patients to protect them from excruciating pain even when it is clear that the time of death will be advanced. The purpose of terminal sedation is to ease the suffering of the patient and comply with her wishes, and the actual cause of death is the administration of heavy doses of lethal sedatives. This same intent and causation may exist when a doctor complies with a patient's request for lethal medication to hasten her death.[15]

Thus, although the differences the majority notes in causation and intent between terminating life support and assisting in suicide support the Court's rejection of the respondents' facial challenge, these distinctions may be inapplicable to particular terminally ill patients and their doctors. Our holding today in *Vacco* v. *Quill* that the Equal Protection Clause is not violated by New York's classification, just like our holding in *Washington* v. *Glucksberg* that the Washington statute is not invalid on its face, does not foreclose the possibility that some applications of the New York statute may impose an intolerable intrusion on the patient's freedom.

There remains room for vigorous debate about the outcome of particular cases that are not necessarily resolved by the opinions announced today. How such cases may be decided will depend on their specific facts. In my judgment, however, it is clear that the so called "unqualified interest in the preservation of human life," *Cruzan,* 497 U.S., at 282, *Glucksberg, ante,* at 24, is not itself sufficient to outweigh the interest in liberty that may justify the only possible means of preserving a dying patient's dignity and alleviating her intolerable suffering.

NOTES

1. *Gregg* v. *Georgia,* 428 U.S. 153 (1976).

2. *Proffitt* v. *Florida,* 428 U.S. 242 (1976).

3. *Jurek* v. *Texas,* 428 U.S. 262 (1976).

4. See, *e.g.*, *Godfrey* v. *Georgia,* 446 U.S. 420 (1980); *Enmund* v. *Florida,* 458 U.S. 782 (1982); *Penry* v. *Lynaugh,* 492 U.S. 302 (1989).

5. See *ante,* at 3, n. 5.

6. If the Court had actually applied the *Salerno* standard in this action, it would have taken only a few paragraphs to identify situations in which the Washington statute could be validly enforced. In *Salerno* itself, the Court would have needed only to look at whether the statute could be constitutionally applied to the arrestees before it; any further analysis would have been superfluous. See Dorf, Facial Challenges to State and Federal Statutes, 46 Stan. L. Rev. 235, 239-240 (1994) (arguing that if the *Salerno* standard were taken literally, a litigant could not succeed in her facial challenge unless she also succeeded in her as applied challenge).

7. In other cases and in other contexts, we have imposed a significantly lesser burden on the challenger. The most lenient standard that we have applied requires the challenger to establish that the invalid applications of a statute "must not only be real, but substantial as well, judged in relation to the statute's plainly legitimate sweep." *Broadrick* v. *Oklahoma,* 413 U.S. 601, 615 (1973). As the Court's opinion demonstrates, Washington's statute prohibiting assisted suicide has a "plainly legitimate sweep." While that demonstration provides a sufficient justification for rejecting respondents' facial challenge, it does not mean that every application of the statute should or will be upheld.

8. "Who casts not up his eye to the sun when it rises? but who takes off his eye from a comet when that breaks out? Who bends not his ear to any bell which upon any occasion rings? but who can remove it from that bell which is passing a piece of himself out of this world? No man is an island, entire of itself; every man is a piece of the continent, a part of the main. If a clod be washed away by the sea, Europe is the less, as well as if a promontory were, as well as if a manor of thy friend's or of thine own were; any man's death diminishes me, because I am involved in mankind; and therefore never send to know for whom the bell tolls; it tolls for thee." J. Donne, Meditation No. 17, Devotions Upon Emergent Occasions 86, 87 (A. Raspa ed. 1987).

9. See 497 U.S., at 332, n. 2.

10. "Neither the Bill of Rights nor the laws of sovereign States create the liberty which the Due Process Clause protects. The relevant constitutional provisions are limitations on the power of the sovereign to infringe on the liberty of the citizen. The relevant state laws either create property rights, or they curtail the freedom of the citizen who must live in an ordered society. Of course, law is essential to the exercise and enjoyment of individual liberty in a complex society. But it is not the source of liberty, and surely not the exclusive source.

"I had thought it self evident that all men were endowed by their Creator with liberty as one of the cardinal unalienable rights. It is that basic freedom which the Due Process Clause protects, rather than the particular rights or privileges conferred by specific laws or regulations." *Meachum* v. *Fano,* 427 U.S. 215, 230 (1976) (Stevens, J., dissenting).

11. "Nancy Cruzan's interest in life, no less than that of any other person, includes an interest in how she will be thought of after her death by those whose opinions mattered to her. There can be no doubt that her life made her dear to her family and to others. How she dies will affect how that life is remembered." *Cruzan* v. *Director, Mo. Dept. of Health*, 497 U.S. 261, 344 (1990) (Stevens, J., dissenting).

"Each of us has an interest in the kind of memories that will survive after death. To that end, individual decisions are often motivated by their impact on others. A member of the kind of family identified in the trial court's findings in this case would likely have not only a normal interest in minimizing the burden that her own illness imposes on others, but also an interest in having their memories of her filled predominantly with thoughts about her past vitality rather than her current condition." *Id.*, at 356.

12. I note that there is evidence that a significant number of physicians support the practice of hastening death in particular situations. A survey published in the New England Journal of Medicine, found that 56% of responding doctors in Michigan preferred legalizing assisted suicide to an explicit ban. Bachman et al., Attitudes of Michigan Physicians and the Public Toward Legalizing Physician Assisted Suicide and Voluntary Euthanasia, 334 New England J. Med. 303-309 (1996). In a survey of Oregon doctors, 60% of the responding doctors supported legalizing assisted suicide for terminally ill patients. See Lee et al., Legalizing Assisted Suicide—Views of Physicians in Oregon, 335 New England J. Med. 310-315 (1996). Another study showed that 12% of physicians polled in Washington State reported that they had been asked by their terminally ill patients for prescriptions to hasten death, and that, in the year prior to the study, 24% of those physicians had complied with such requests. See Back, Wallace, Starks, & Perlman, Physician Assisted Suicide and Euthanasia in Washington State, 275 JAMA 919-925 (1996); see also Doukas, Waterhouse, Gorenflo, & Seld, Attitudes and Behaviors on Physician Assisted Death: A Study of Michigan Oncologists, 13 J. Clinical Oncology 1055 (1995) (reporting that 18% of responding Michigan oncologists reported active participation in assisted suicide); Slome, Moulton, Huffine, Gorter, & Abrams, Physicians' Attitudes Toward Assisted Suicide in AIDS, 5 J. Acquired Immune Deficiency Syndromes 712 (1992) (reporting that 24% of responding physicians who treat AIDS patients would likely grant a patient's request for assistance in hastening death).

13. See *Vacco* v. *Quill, ante,* at 1, nn. 1 and 2.

14. The American Medical Association recognized this distinction when it supported Nancy Cruzan and continues to recognize this distinction in its support of the States in these cases.

15. If a doctor prescribes lethal drugs to be self administered by the patient, it not at all clear that the physician's intent is that the patient "be made dead," *ante,* at 7 (internal quotation marks omitted). Many patients prescribed lethal medications never actually take them; they merely acquire some sense of control in the process of dying that the availability of those medications provides. See Back, *supra* n. 12, at 922; see also Quill, 324 New England J. Med., at 693

(describing how some patients fear death less when they feel they have the option of physician assisted suicide).

Supreme Court of the United States

No. 96-110

WASHINGTON ET AL., PETITIONERS *v.* HAROLD GLUCKSBERG
ET AL.

ON WRIT OF CERTIORARI TO THE UNITED STATES COURT OF
APPEALS FOR THE NINTH CIRCUIT

[JUNE 26, 1997]

Justice Souter, concurring in the judgment.

Three terminally ill individuals and four physicians who sometimes treat terminally ill patients brought this challenge to the Washington statute making it a crime "knowingly . . . [to] aid another person to attempt suicide," Wash. Rev. Code §9A.36.060 (1994), claiming on behalf of both patients and physicians that it would violate substantive due process to enforce the statute against a doctor who acceded to a dying patient's request for a drug to be taken by the patient to commit suicide. The question is whether the statute sets up one of those "arbitrary impositions" or "purposeless restraints" at odds with the Due Process Clause of the Fourteenth Amendment. *Poe* v. *Ullman*, 367 U.S. 497, 543 (1961) (Harlan, J., dissenting). I conclude that the statute's application to the doctors has not been shown to be unconstitutional, but I write separately to give my reasons for analyzing the substantive due process claims as I do, and for rejecting this one.

Although the terminally ill original parties have died during the pendency of this case, the four physicians who remain as respondents here[1] continue to request declaratory and injunctive relief for their own benefit in discharging their obligations to other dying patients who request their help.[2] See, *e.g., Southern Pacific Terminal Co.* v. *ICC*, 219 U.S. 498, 515 (1911) (question was capable of repetition yet evading review). The case reaches us on an order granting summary judgment, and we must take as true the undisputed allegations that each of the patients was mentally competent and terminally ill, and that each made a knowing and voluntary choice to ask a doctor to prescribe "medications . . . to be self administered for the purpose of hastening . . . death." Complaint ¶ 2.3. The State does not dispute that each faced a passage to death more agonizing both mentally and physically, and more protracted over time, than death by suicide with a physician's help, or that each would have chosen such a suicide for the sake of personal dignity, apart even from relief from pain. Each doctor in this case claims to encounter patients like the original plaintiffs who have died, that is, mentally competent, terminally ill, and seeking medical help in "the voluntary self termination of life." *Id.*, at ¶ 2.5-2.8. While there may be no unanimity on the physician's professional obligation in such circumstances, I accept here respondents' representation that providing such patients with prescriptions for drugs that go beyond pain relief to hasten death would, in these circumstances, be consistent with standards of medical practice. Hence, I take it to be true, as respondents say, that the Washington statute prevents the exercise of a physician's "best professional judgment to prescribe medications to [such] patients in dosages that would enable them to act to hasten their own deaths." *Id.*, at 2.6; see also App. 35-37, 49-51, 55-57, 73-75.

In their brief to this Court, the doctors claim not that they ought to have a right generally to hasten patients' imminent deaths, but only to help patients who have made "personal decisions regarding their own bodies, medical care, and, fundamentally, the future course of their lives," Brief for Respondents 12, and who have concluded responsibly and with substantial justification that the brief and anguished remainders of their lives have lost virtually all value to them. Respondents fully embrace the notion that the State must be free to impose reasonable regulations on such physician assistance to ensure that the patients they assist are indeed among the competent and terminally ill and that each has made a free and informed choice in seeking to obtain and use a fatal drug. Complaint 3.2; App. 28-41.

In response, the State argues that the interest asserted by the doctors is beyond constitutional recognition because it has no deep roots in our history and traditions. Brief for Petitioners 21-25. But even aside from that, without disputing that the patients here were competent and terminally ill, the State insists that recognizing the legitimacy of doctors' assistance of their patients as contemplated here would entail a number of adverse consequences that the Washington Legislature was entitled to forestall. The nub of this part of the State's argument is not that such patients are constitutionally undeserving of relief on their own account, but that any attempt to confine a right of physician assistance to the circumstances presented by these doctors is likely to fail. *Id.*, at 34-35, 44-47.

First, the State argues that the right could not be confined to the terminally ill. Even assuming a fixed definition of that term, the State observes that it is not always possible to say with certainty how long a person may live. *Id.*, at 34. It asserts that "[t]here is no principled basis on which [the right] can be limited to the prescription of medication for terminally ill patients to administer to themselves" when the right's justifying principle is as broad as "'merciful termination of suffering.'" *Id.*, at 45 (citing Y. Kamisar, Are Laws Against Assisted Suicide Unconstitutional?, Hastings Center Report 32, 36-37 (May June 1993)). Second, the State argues that the right could not be confined to the mentally competent, observing that a person's competence cannot always be assessed with certainty, Brief for Petitioners 34, and suggesting further that no principled distinction is possible between a competent patient acting independently and a patient acting through a duly appointed and competent surrogate, *id.*, at 46. Next, according to the State, such a right might entail a right to or at least merge in practice into "other forms of life ending assistance," such as euthanasia. *Id.*, at 46-47. Finally, the State believes that a right to physician assistance could not easily be distinguished from a right to assistance from others, such as friends, family, and other health care workers. *Id.*, at 47. The State thus argues that recognition of the substantive due process right at issue here would jeopardize the lives of others outside the class defined by the doctors' claim, creating risks of irresponsible suicides and euthanasia, whose dangers are concededly within the State's authority to address.

When the physicians claim that the Washington law deprives them of a right falling within the scope of liberty that the Fourteenth Amendment guarantees against denial without due process of law,[3] they are not claiming some sort of procedural defect in the process through which the statute has been enacted or is administered. Their claim, rather, is that the State has no substantively adequate justification for barring the assistance sought by the patient and sought to be offered by the physician. Thus, we are dealing with a claim to one of those rights sometimes described as rights of substantive due process and sometimes as unenumerated rights, in view of the breadth and indeterminacy of the "due process" serving as the claim's textual basis. The doctors accordingly arouse the skepticism of those who find the Due Process Clause an unduly vague or oxymoronic warrant for judicial review of substantive state law, just as they also invoke two centuries of American constitutional practice in recognizing unenumerated, substantive limits on governmental action. Although this practice has neither rested on any single textual basis nor expressed a consistent theory (or, before *Poe* v. *Ullman*, a much articulated one), a brief overview of its history is instructive on two counts. The persistence of substantive due process in our cases points to the legitimacy of the modern justification for such judicial review found in Justice Harlan's dissent in *Poe*,[4] on which I will dwell further on, while the acknowledged failures of some of these cases point with caution to the difficulty raised by the present claim.

Before the ratification of the Fourteenth Amendment, substantive constitutional review resting on a theory of unenumerated rights occurred largely in the state courts applying state constitutions that commonly contained either due process clauses like that of the Fifth Amendment (and later the Fourteenth) or the textual antecedents of such clauses, repeating Magna Carta's guarantee of "the law of the land."[5] On the basis of such clauses, or of general principles untethered to specific constitutional language, state courts evaluated the constitutionality of a wide range of statutes.

Thus, a Connecticut court approved a statute legitimating a class of previous illegitimate marriages, as falling within the terms of the "social compact," while making clear its power to review constitutionality in those terms. *Goshen* v. *Stonington*, 4 Conn. 209, 225-226 (1822). In the same period, a specialized court of equity, created under a Tennessee statute solely to hear cases brought by the state bank against its debtors, found its own authorization unconstitutional as "partial" legislation violating the state constitution's "law of the land" clause. *Bank of the State* v. *Cooper*, 2 Yerg. 599, 602-608 (Tenn. 1831) (Green, J.); *id.*, at 613-615 (Peck, J.); *id.*, at 618-623 (Kennedy, J.). And the middle of the 19th century brought the famous *Wynehamer* case, invalidating a statute purporting to render possession of liquor immediately illegal except when kept for narrow, specified purposes, the state court finding the statute inconsistent with the state's due process clause. *Wynehamer* v. *People*, 13 N.Y. 378, 486-487 (1856). The statute was deemed an excessive threat to the "fundamental rights of the citizen" to property. *Id.*, at 398 (Comstock, J.). See generally, E. Corwin, Liberty Against Government 58-115 (1948) (discussing substantive due process in the state courts before the Civil War); T. Cooley, Constitutional Limitations *85-*129, *351-*397.

Even in this early period, however, this Court anticipated the developments that would presage both the Civil War and the ratification of the Fourteenth Amendment, by making it clear on several occasions that it too had no doubt of the judiciary's power to strike down legislation that conflicted with important but unenumerated principles of American government. In most such instances, after declaring its power to invalidate what it might find inconsistent with rights of liberty and property, the Court nevertheless went on to uphold the legislative acts under review. See, *e.g.*, *Wilkinson* v. *Leland*, 2 Pet. 627, 656-661 (1829); *Calder* v. *Bull*, 3 Dall. 386, 386-395 (1798) (opinion of Chase, J.); see also *Corfield* v. *Coryell*, 6 F. Cas. 546, 550-552 (No. 3,230) (1823). But in *Fletcher* v. *Peck*, 6 Cranch 87 (1810), the Court went further. It struck down an act of the Georgia legislature that purported to rescind a sale of public land *ab initio* and reclaim title for the State, and so deprive subsequent, good faith purchasers of property conveyed by the original grantees. The Court rested the invalidation on alternative sources of authority: the specific prohibitions against bills of attainder, *ex post-facto* laws, laws impairing contracts in Article I, § 10 of the Constitution; and "general principles which are common to our free institutions," by which Chief Justice Marshall meant that a simple deprivation of property by the State could not be an authentically "legislative" act. *Fletcher*, 6 Cranch, at 135-139.

Fletcher was not, though, the most telling early example of such review. For its most salient instance in this Court before the adoption of the Fourteenth Amendment was, of course, the case that the Amendment would in due course overturn, *Dred Scott* v. *Sandford*, 19 How. 393 (1857). Unlike *Fletcher*, *Dred Scott* was textually based on a due process clause (in the Fifth Amendment, applicable to the national government), and it was in reliance on that clause's protection of property that the Court invalidated the Missouri Compromise. 19 How., at 449-452. This substantive protection of an owner's property in a slave taken to the territories was traced to the absence of any enumerated power to affect that property granted to the Congress by Article I of the Constitution, *id.*, at 451-452, the implication being that the government had no legitimate interest that could support the earlier congressional compromise. The ensuing judgment of history needs no recounting here.

After the ratification of the Fourteenth Amendment, with its guarantee of due process protection against the States, interpretation of the words "liberty" and "property" as used in due process clauses became a sustained enterprise, with the Court generally describing the due process criterion in converse terms of reasonableness or arbitrariness. That standard is fairly traceable to Justice Bradley's dissent in the *Slaughter House Cases*, 16 Wall. 36 (1873), in which he said that a person's right to choose a calling was an element of liberty (as the calling, once chosen, was an aspect of property) and declared that the liberty and property protected by due process are not truly recognized if such rights may be "arbitrarily assailed," *id.*, at 116.[6] After that, opinions comparable to those that preceded *Dred Scott* expressed willingness to review legislative action for consistency with the Due Process Clause even as they upheld the laws in question. See, *e.g., Bartemeyer* v. *Iowa,* 18 Wall. 129, 133-135 (1874); *Munn* v. *Illinois,* 94 U.S. 113, 123-135 (1877); *Railroad Comm'n Cases,* 116 U.S. 307, 331 (1886); *Mugler* v. *Kansas,* 123 U.S. 623, 659-670 (1887). See generally Corwin, Liberty Against Government, at 121-136 (surveying the Court's early Fourteenth Amendment cases and finding little dissent from the general principle that the Due Process Clause authorized judicial review of substantive statutes).

The theory became serious, however, beginning with *Allgeyer* v. *Louisiana,* 165 U.S. 578 (1897), where the Court invalidated a Louisiana statute for excessive interference with Fourteenth Amendment liberty to contract, *id.*, at 588-593, and offered a substantive interpretation of "liberty," that in the aftermath of the so called Lochner Era has been scaled back in some respects, but expanded in others, and never repudiated in principle. The Court said that Fourteenth Amendment liberty includes "the right of the citizen to be free in the enjoyment of all his faculties; to be free to use them in all lawful ways; to live and work where he will; to earn his livelihood by any lawful calling; to pursue any livelihood or avocation; and for that purpose to enter into all contracts which may be proper, necessary and essential to his carrying out to a successful conclusion the purposes above mentioned." *Id.*, at 589. "[W]e do not intend to hold that in no such case can the State exercise its police power," the Court added, but "[w]hen and how far such power may be legitimately exercised with regard to these subjects must be left for determination to each case as it arises." *Id.*, at 590.

Although this principle was unobjectionable, what followed for a season was, in the realm of economic legislation, the echo of *Dred Scott. Allgeyer* was succeeded within a decade by *Lochner* v. *New York,* 198 U.S. 45 (1905), and the era to which that case gave its name, famous now for striking down as arbitrary various sorts of economic regulations that post-New Deal courts have uniformly thought constitutionally sound. Compare, *e.g., id.*, at 62 (finding New York's maximum hours law for bakers "unreasonable and entirely arbitrary") and *Adkins* v. *Children's Hospital of D. C.,* 261 U.S. 525, 559 (1923) (holding a minimum wage law "so clearly the product of a naked, arbitrary exercise of power that it cannot be allowed to stand under the Constitution of the United States") with *West Coast Hotel Co.* v. *Parrish,* 300 U.S. 379, 391 (1937) (overruling *Adkins* and approving a minimum wage law on the principle that "regulation which is reasonable in relation to its subject and is adopted in the interests of the community is due process"). As the parentheticals here suggest, while the cases in the *Lochner* line routinely invoked a correct standard of constitutional arbitrariness review, they harbored the spirit of *Dred Scott* in their absolutist implementation of the standard they espoused.

Even before the deviant economic due process cases had been repudiated, however, the more durable precursors of modern substantive due process were reaffirming this Court's obligation to conduct arbitrariness review, beginning with *Meyer* v. *Nebraska,* 262 U.S. 390 (1923). Without referring to any specific guarantee of the Bill of Rights, the Court invoked precedents from the *Slaughter House Cases* through *Adkins* to declare that the Fourteenth Amendment protected "the right of the individual to contract, to engage in any of the common occupations of life, to acquire useful knowledge, to marry, establish a home and bring up children, to worship God according to the dictates of his own conscience, and generally to enjoy those privileges long recognized at common law as essential to the orderly pursuit of happiness by free men." *Id.,* at 399. The Court then held that the same Fourteenth Amendment liberty included a teacher's right to teach and the rights of parents to direct their children's education without unreasonable interference by the States, *id.,* at 400, with the result that Nebraska's prohibition on the teaching of foreign languages in the lower grades was, "arbitrary and without reasonable relation to any end within the competency of the State," *id.,* at 403. See also *Pierce* v. *Society of Sisters,* 268 U.S. 510, 534-536 (1925) (finding that a statute that all but outlawed private schools lacked any "reasonable relation to some purpose within the competency of the State"); *Palko* v. *Connecticut,* 302 U.S. 319, 327-238 (1937) ("even in the field of substantive rights and duties the legislative judgment, if oppressive and arbitrary, may be overridden by the courts"; "Is that [injury] to which the statute has subjected [the appellant] a hardship so acute and shocking that our polity will not endure it? Does it violate those fundamental principles of liberty and justice which lie at the base of all our civil and political institutions?") (citation and internal quotation marks omitted).

After *Meyer* and *Pierce,* two further opinions took the major steps that lead to the modern law. The first was not even in a due process case but one about equal protection, *Skinner* v. *Oklahoma ex rel. Williamson,* 316 U.S. 535 (1942), where the Court emphasized the "fundamental" nature of individual choice about procreation and so foreshadowed not only the later prominence of procreation as a subject of liberty protection, but the corresponding standard of "strict scrutiny," in this Court's Fourteenth Amendment law. See *id.,* at 541. *Skinner,* that is, added decisions regarding procreation to the list of liberties recognized in *Meyer* and *Pierce* and loosely suggested, as a gloss on their standard of arbitrariness, a judicial obligation to scrutinize any impingement on such an important interest with heightened care. In so doing, it suggested a point that Justice Harlan would develop, that the kind and degree of justification that a sensitive judge would demand of a State would depend on the importance of the interest being asserted by the individual. *Poe,* 367 U.S., at 543.

The second major opinion leading to the modern doctrine was Justice Harlan's *Poe* dissent just cited, the conclusion of which was adopted in *Griswold* v. *Connecticut,* 381 U.S. 478 (1965), and the authority of which was acknowledged in *Planned Parenthood of Southeastern Pa.* v. *Casey,* 505 U.S. 833 (1992). See also n. 4, *supra.* The dissent is important for three things that point to our responsibilities today. The first is Justice Harlan's respect for the tradition of substantive due process review itself, and his acknowledgement of the Judiciary's obligation to carry it on. For two centuries American courts, and for much of that time this Court, have thought it necessary to provide some degree of review over the substantive content of legislation under constitutional standards of textual breadth. The obligation was understood before *Dred Scott* and has continued after the repudiation of *Lochner*'s progeny, most notably on the subjects of segregation in public education, *Bolling* v. *Sharpe*, 347 U.S. 497, 500 (1954), interracial marriage, *Loving* v. *Virginia*, 388 U.S. 1, 12 (1967), marital privacy and contraception, *Carey* v. *Population Services Int'l*, 431 U.S. 678, 684-691 (1977), *Griswold* v. *Connecticut, supra*, at 481-486, abortion, *Planned Parenthood of Southeastern Pa.* v. *Casey*, 505 U.S. 833, 849, 869-879 (1992) (joint opinion of O'Connor, Kennedy, and Souter, JJ.), *Roe* v. *Wade*, 410 U.S. 113, 152-166 (1973), personal control of medical treatment, *Cruzan* v. *Director, Mo. Dept. of Health*, 497 U.S. 261, 287-289 (1990) (O'Connor, J., concurring); *id.*, at 302 (Brennan, J., dissenting); *id.*, at 331 (Stevens, J., dissenting); see also *id.*, at 278 (majority opinion), and physical confinement, *Foucha* v. *Louisiana*, 504 U.S. 71, 80-83 (1992). This enduring tradition of American constitutional practice is, in Justice Harlan's view, nothing more than what is required by the judicial authority and obligation to construe constitutional text and review legislation for conformity to that text. See *Marbury* v. *Madison*, 1 Cranch 137 (1803). Like many judges who preceded him and many who followed, he found it impossible to construe the text of due process without recognizing substantive, and not merely procedural, limitations. "Were due process merely a procedural safeguard it would fail to reach those situations where the deprivation of life, liberty or property was accomplished by legislation which by operating in the future could, given even the fairest possible procedure in application to individuals, nevertheless destroy the enjoyment of all three." *Poe*, 367 U.S., at 541.[7] The text of the Due Process Clause thus imposes nothing less than an obligation to give substantive content to the words "liberty" and "due process of law."

Following the first point of the *Poe* dissent, on the necessity to engage in the sort of examination we conduct today, the dissent's second and third implicitly address those cases, already noted, that are now condemned with virtual unanimity as disastrous mistakes of substantive due process review. The second of the dissent's lessons is a reminder that the business of such review is not the identification of extratextual absolutes but scrutiny of a legislative resolution (perhaps unconscious) of clashing principles, each quite possibly worthy in and of itself, but each to be weighed within the history of our values as a people. It is a comparison of the relative strengths of opposing claims that informs the judicial task, not a deduction from some first premise. Thus informed, judicial review still has no warrant to substitute one reasonable resolution of the contending positions for another, but authority to supplant the balance already struck between the contenders only when it falls outside the realm of the reasonable. Part III, below, deals with this second point, and also with the dissent's third, which takes the form of an object lesson in the explicit attention to detail that is no less essential to the intellectual discipline of substantive due process review than an understanding of the basic need to account for the two sides in the controversy and to respect legislation within the zone of reasonableness.

My understanding of unenumerated rights in the wake of the *Poe* dissent and subsequent cases avoids the absolutist failing of many older cases without embracing the opposite pole of equating reasonableness with past practice described at a very specific level. See *Planned Parenthood of Southeastern Pa.* v. *Casey*, 505 U.S. 833, 847-849 (1992). That understanding begins with a concept of "ordered liberty," *Poe*, 367 U. S., at 549 (Harlan, J.); see also *Griswold*, 381 U.S., at 500, comprising a continuum of rights to be free from "arbitrary impositions and purposeless restraints," *Poe*, 367 U.S., at 543 (Harlan, J., dissenting).

"Due Process has not been reduced to any formula; its content cannot be determined by reference to any code. The best that can be said is that through the course of this Court's decisions it has represented the balance which our Nation, built upon postulates of respect for the liberty of the individual, has struck between that liberty and the demands of organized society. If the supplying of content to this Constitutional concept has of necessity been a rational process, it certainly has not been one where judges have felt free to roam where unguided speculation might take them. The balance of which I speak is the balance struck by this country, having regard to what history teaches are the traditions from which it developed as well as the traditions from which it broke. That tradition is a living thing. A decision of this Court which radically departs from it could not long survive, while a decision which builds on what has survived is likely to be sound. No formula could serve as a substitute, in this area, for judgment and restraint." *Id., at* 542.

See also *Moore* v. *East Cleveland*, 431 U.S. 494, 503 (1977) (plurality opinion of Powell, J.) ("Appropriate limits on substantive due process come not from drawing arbitrary lines but rather from careful 'respect for the teachings of history [and] solid recognition of the basic values that underlie our society' ") (quoting *Griswold*, 481 U.S., at 501 (Harlan, J., concurring)).

After the *Poe* dissent, as before it, this enforceable concept of liberty would bar statutory impositions even at relatively trivial levels when governmental restraints are undeniably irrational as unsupported by any imaginable rationale. See, *e.g., United States* v. *Carolene Products Co.*, 304 U.S. 144, 152 (1938) (economic legislation "not . . . unconstitutional unless . . . facts . . . preclude the assumption that it rests upon some rational basis"); see also *Poe*, 367 U.S., at 545, 548 (Harlan, J., dissenting) (referring to usual "presumption of constitutionality" and ordinary test "going merely to the plausibility of [a statute's] underlying rationale"). Such instances are suitably rare. The claims of arbitrariness that mark almost all instances of unenumerated substantive rights are those resting on "certain interests requiring particularly careful scrutiny of the state needs asserted to justify their abridgment. Cf. *Skinner* v. *Oklahoma* [*ex rel. Williamson*, 316 U.S. 535 (1942)]; *Bolling* v. *Sharpe*, [347 U.S. 497 (1954)]," *id.*, at 543; that is, interests in liberty sufficiently important to be judged "fundamental," *id.*, at 548; see also *id.*, at 541 (citing *Corfield* v. *Coryell*, 4 Wash. C.C. 371, 380 (CC ED Pa. 1825)). In the face of an interest this powerful a State may not rest on threshold rationality or a presumption of constitutionality, but may prevail only on the ground of an interest sufficiently compelling to place within the realm of the reasonable a refusal to recognize the individual right asserted. *Poe, supra*, at 548 (Harlan, J., dissenting) (an "enactment involving . . . a most fundamental aspect of 'liberty' . . . [is] subject to 'strict scrutiny' ") (quoting *Skinner* v. *Oklahoma ex rel. Williamson*, 316 U.S., at 541);[8] *Reno* v. *Flores*, 507 U.S. 292, 301-302 (1993) (reaffirming that due process "forbids the government to infringe certain 'fundamental' liberty interests . . . unless the infringement is narrowly tailored to serve a compelling state interest").[9]

This approach calls for a court to assess the relative "weights" or dignities of the contending interests, and to this extent the judicial method is familiar to the common law. Common law method is subject, however, to two important constraints in the hands of a court engaged in substantive due process review. First, such a court is bound to confine the values that it recognizes to those truly deserving constitutional stature, either to those expressed in constitutional text, or those exemplified by "the traditions from which [the Nation] developed," or revealed by contrast with "the traditions from which it broke." *Poe*, 367 U.S., at 542 (Harlan, J., dissenting). "'We may not draw on our merely personal and private notions and disregard the limits . . . derived from considerations that are fused in the whole nature of our judicial process . . . [,] considerations deeply rooted in reason and in the compelling traditions of the legal profession.'" *Id.*, at 544-545 (quoting *Rochin* v. *California*, 342 U.S. 165, 170-171 (1952)); see also *Palko* v. *Connecticut*, 302 U.S., at 325 (looking to "'principle[s] of justice so rooted in the traditions and conscience of our people as to be ranked as fundamental'") (quoting *Snyder* v. *Massachusetts*, 291 U.S. 97, 105 (1934)).

The second constraint, again, simply reflects the fact that constitutional review, not judicial lawmaking, is a court's business here. The weighing or valuing of contending interests in this sphere is only the first step, forming the basis for determining whether the statute in question falls inside or outside the zone of what is reasonable in the way it resolves the conflict between the interests of state and individual. See, *e.g., Poe, supra*, at 553 (Harlan, J., dissenting); *Youngberg* v. *Romeo*, 457 U.S. 307, 320-321 (1982). It is no justification for judicial intervention merely to identify a reasonable resolution of contending values that differs from the terms of the legislation under review. It is only when the legislation's justifying principle, critically valued, is so far from being commensurate with the individual interest as to be arbitrarily or pointlessly applied that the statute must give way. Only if this standard points against the statute can the individual claimant be said to have a constitutional right. See *Cruzan* v. *Director, Mo. Dept. of Health*, 497 U.S., at 279 ("Determining that a person has a 'liberty interest' under the Due Process Clause does not end the inquiry; 'whether [the individual's] constitutional rights have been violated must be determined by balancing his liberty interests against the relevant state interests'") (quoting *Youngberg* v. *Romeo, supra*, at 321).[10]

The *Poe* dissent thus reminds us of the nature of review for reasonableness or arbitrariness and the limitations entailed by it. But the opinion cautions against the repetition of past error in another way as well, more by its example than by any particular statement of constitutional method: it reminds us that the process of substantive review by reasoned judgment, *Poe*, 367 U.S., at 542-544, is one of close criticism going to the details of the opposing interests and to their relationships with the historically recognized principles that lend them weight or value.

Although the *Poe* dissent disclaims the possibility of any general formula for due process analysis (beyond the basic analytic structure just described), see *id.*, at 542, 544, Justice Harlan of course assumed that adjudication under the Due Process Clauses is like any other instance of judgment dependent on common law method, being more or less persuasive according to the usual canons of critical discourse. See also *Casey*, 505 U.S., at 849 ("The inescapable fact is that adjudication of substantive due process claims may call upon the Court in interpreting the Constitution to exercise that same capacity which by tradition courts always have exercised: reasoned judgment"). When identifying and assessing the competing interests of liberty and authority, for example, the breadth of expression that a litigant or a judge selects in stating the competing principles will have much to do with the outcome and may be dispositive. As in any process of rational argumentation, we recognize that when a generally accepted principle is challenged, the broader the attack the less likely it is to succeed. The principle's defenders will, indeed, often try to characterize any challenge as just such a broadside, perhaps by couching the defense as if a broadside attack had occurred. So the Court in *Dred Scott* treated prohibition of slavery in the Territories as nothing less than a general assault on the concept of property. See *Dred Scott v. Sandford*, 19 How., at 449-452.

Just as results in substantive due process cases are tied to the selections of statements of the competing interests, the acceptability of the results is a function of the good reasons for the selections made. It is here that the value of common law method becomes apparent, for the usual thinking of the common law is suspicious of the all or nothing analysis that tends to produce legal petrification instead of an evolving boundary between the domains of old principles. Common law method tends to pay respect instead to detail, seeking to understand old principles afresh by new examples and new counterexamples. The "tradition is a living thing," *Poe*, 367 U.S., at 542 (Harlan, J., dissenting), albeit one that moves by moderate steps carefully taken. "The decision of an apparently novel claim must depend on grounds which follow closely on well accepted principles and criteria. The new decision must take its place in relation to what went before and further [cut] a channel for what is to come." *Id.*, at 544 (Harlan, J., dissenting) (internal quotation marks omitted). Exact analysis and characterization of any due process claim is critical to the method and to the result.

So, in *Poe*, Justice Harlan viewed it as essential to the plaintiffs' claimed right to use contraceptives that they sought to do so within the privacy of the marital bedroom. This detail in fact served two crucial and complementary functions, and provides a lesson for today. It rescued the individuals' claim from a breadth that would have threatened all state regulation of contraception or intimate relations; extramarital intimacy, no matter how privately practiced, was outside the scope of the right Justice Harlan would have recognized in that case. See *id.*, at 552-553. It was, moreover, this same restriction that allowed the interest to be valued as an aspect of a broader liberty to be free from all unreasonable intrusions into the privacy of the home and the family life within it, a liberty exemplified in constitutional provisions such as the Third and Fourth Amendments, in prior decisions of the Court involving unreasonable intrusions into the home and family life, and in the then prevailing status of marriage as the sole lawful locus of intimate relations. *Id.*, at 548, 551.[11] The individuals' interest was therefore at its peak in *Poe,* because it was supported by a principle that distinguished of its own force between areas in which government traditionally had regulated (sexual relations outside of marriage) and those in which it had not (private marital intimacies), and thus was broad enough to cover the claim at hand without being so broad as to be shot through by exceptions.

On the other side of the balance, the State's interest in *Poe* was not fairly characterized simply as preserving sexual morality, or doing so by regulating contraceptive devices. Just as some of the earlier cases went astray by speaking without nuance of individual interests in property or autonomy to contract for labor, so the State's asserted interest in *Poe* was not immune to distinctions turning (at least potentially) on the precise purpose being pursued and the collateral consequences of the means chosen, see *id.,* at 547-548. It was assumed that the State might legitimately enforce limits on the use of contraceptives through laws regulating divorce and annulment, or even through its tax policy, *ibid.,* but not necessarily be justified in criminalizing the same practice in the marital bedroom, which would entail the consequence of authorizing state enquiry into the intimate relations of a married couple who chose to close their door, *id.,* at 548-549. See also *Casey,* 505 U.S., at 869 (strength of State's interest in potential life varies depending on precise context and character of regulation pursuing that interest).

The same insistence on exactitude lies behind questions, in current terminology, about the proper level of generality at which to analyze claims and counter claims, and the demand for fitness and proper tailoring of a restrictive statute is just another way of testing the legitimacy of the generality at which the government sets up its justification.[12] We may therefore classify Justice Harlan's example of proper analysis in any of these ways: as applying concepts of normal critical reasoning, as pointing to the need to attend to the levels of generality at which countervailing interests are stated, or as examining the concrete application of principles for fitness with their own ostensible justifications. But whatever the categories in which we place the dissent's example, it stands in marked contrast to earlier cases whose reasoning was marked by comparatively less discrimination, and it points to the importance of evaluating the claims of the parties now before us with comparable detail. For here we are faced with an individual claim not to a right on the part of just anyone to help anyone else commit suicide under any circumstances, but to the right of a narrow class to help others also in a narrow class under a set of limited circumstances. And the claimants are met with the State's assertion, among others, that rights of such narrow scope cannot be recognized without jeopardy to individuals whom the State may concededly protect through its regulations.

Respondents claim that a patient facing imminent death, who anticipates physical suffering and indignity, and is capable of responsible and voluntary choice, should have a right to a physician's assistance in providing counsel and drugs to be administered by the patient to end life promptly. Complaint 3.1. They accordingly claim that a physician must have the corresponding right to provide such aid, contrary to the provisions of Wash. Rev. Code §9A.36.060

(1994). I do not understand the argument to rest on any assumption that rights either to suicide or to assistance in committing it are historically based as such. Respondents, rather, acknowledge the prohibition of each historically, but rely on the fact that to a substantial extent the State has repudiated that history. The result of this, respondents say, is to open the door to claims of such a patient to be accorded one of the options open to those with different, traditionally cognizable claims to autonomy in deciding how their bodies and minds should be treated. They seek the option to obtain the services of a physician to give them the benefit of advice and medical help, which is said to enjoy a tradition so strong and so devoid of specifically countervailing state concern that denial of a physician's help in these circumstances is arbitrary when physicians are generally free to advise and aid those who exercise other rights to bodily autonomy.

The dominant western legal codes long condemned suicide and treated either its attempt or successful accomplishment as a crime, the one subjecting the individual to penalties, the other penalizing his survivors by designating the suicide's property as forfeited to the government. See 4 W. Blackstone, Commentaries *188-*189 (commenting that English law considered suicide to be "ranked . . . among the highest crimes" and deemed persuading another to commit suicide to be murder); see generally Marzen, O'Dowd, Crone, & Balch, Suicide: A Constitutional Right?, 24 Duquense L. Rev. 1, 56-63 (1985). While suicide itself has generally not been considered a punishable crime in the United States, largely because the common law punishment of forfeiture was rejected as improperly penalizing an innocent family, see *id.*, at 98-99, most States have consistently punished the act of assisting a suicide as either a common law or statutory crime and some continue to view suicide as an unpunishable crime. See generally *id.*, at 67-100, 148-242.[13] Criminal prohibitions on such assistance remain widespread, as exemplified in the Washington statute in question here.[14]

The principal significance of this history in the State of Washington, according to respondents, lies in its repudiation of the old tradition to the extent of eliminating the criminal suicide prohibitions. Respondents do not argue that the State's decision goes further, to imply that the State has repudiated any legitimate claim to discourage suicide or to limit its encouragement. The reasons for the decriminalization, after all, may have had more to do with difficulties of law enforcement than with a shift in the value ascribed to life in various circumstances or in the perceived legitimacy of taking one's own. See, *e.g.*, Kamisar, Physician Assisted Suicide: The Last Bridge to Active Voluntary Euthanasia, in Euthanasia Examined 225, 229 (J. Keown ed. 1995); CeloCruz, Aid in Dying: Should We Decriminalize Physician Assisted Suicide and Physician Committed Euthanasia?, 18 Am. J. L. & Med. 369, 375 (1992); Marzen, O'Dowd, Crone, & Balch 24 Duquesne L. Rev. *supra*, at 98-99. Thus it may indeed make sense for the State to take its hands off suicide as such, while continuing to prohibit the sort of assistance that would make its commission easier. See, *e.g.*, American Law Institute, Model Penal Code §210.5, Comment 5 (1980). Decriminalization does not, then, imply the existence of a constitutional liberty interest in suicide as such; it simply opens the door to the assertion of a cognizable liberty interest in bodily integrity and associated medical care that would otherwise have been inapposite so long as suicide, as well as assisting a suicide, was a criminal offense.

This liberty interest in bodily integrity was phrased in a general way by then Judge Cardozo when he said, "every human being of adult years and sound mind has a right to determine what shall be done with his own body" in relation to his medical needs. *Schloendorff* v. *Society of New York Hospital,* 211 N.Y. 125, 129, 105 N.E. 92, 93 (1914). The familiar examples of this right derive from the common law of battery and include the right to be free from medical invasions into the body, *Cruzan* v. *Director, Mo. Dept. of Health,* 497 U.S., at 269-279, as well as a right generally to resist enforced medication, see *Washington* v. *Harper,* 494 U.S. 210, 221-222, 229 (1990). Thus "it is settled now . . . that the Constitution places limits on a State's right to interfere with a person's most basic decisions about . . . bodily integrity." *Casey,* 505 U. S., at 849 (citations omitted); see also *Cruzan,* 497 U.S., at 278; *id.,* at 288 (O'Connor, J., concurring); *Washington* v. *Harper, supra,* at 221-222; *Winston* v. *Lee,* 470 U.S. 753, 761-762 (1985); *Rochin* v. *California,* 342 U.S., at 172. Constitutional recognition of the right to bodily integrity underlies the assumed right, good against the State, to require physicians to terminate artificial life support, *Cruzan, supra,* at 279 ("we assume that the United States Constitution would grant a competent person a constitutionally protected right to refuse lifesaving hydration and nutrition"), and the affirmative right to obtain medical intervention to cause abortion, see *Casey, supra,* at 857, 896; cf. *Roe* v. *Wade,* 410 U.S., at 153.

It is, indeed, in the abortion cases that the most telling recognitions of the importance of bodily integrity and the concomitant tradition of medical assistance have occurred. In *Roe* v. *Wade,* the plaintiff contended that the Texas statute making it criminal for any person to "procure an abortion," *id.,* at 117, for a pregnant woman was unconstitutional insofar as it prevented her from "terminating her pregnancy by an abortion 'performed by a competent, licensed physician, under safe, clinical conditions,'" *id.,* at 120, and in striking down the statute we stressed the importance of the relationship between patient and physician, see *id.,* at 153, 156.

The analogies between the abortion cases and this one are several. Even though the State has a legitimate interest in discouraging abortion, see *Casey,* 505 U.S., at 871 (joint opinion of O'Connor, Kennedy, and Souter, JJ.) *Roe,* 410 U.S., at 162, the Court recognized a woman's right to a physician's counsel and care. Like the decision to commit suicide, the decision to abort potential life can be made irresponsibly and under the influence of others, and yet the Court has held in the abortion cases that physicians are fit assistants. Without physician assistance in abortion, the woman's right would have too often amounted to nothing more than a right to self mutilation, and without a physician to assist in the suicide of the dying, the patient's right will often be confined to crude methods of causing death, most shocking and painful to the decedent's survivors.

There is, finally, one more reason for claiming that a physician's assistance here would fall within the accepted tradition of medical care in our society, and the abortion cases are only the most obvious illustration of the further point. While the Court has held that the performance of abortion procedures can be restricted to physicians, the Court's opinion in *Roe* recognized the doctors' role in yet another way. For, in the course of holding that the decision to perform an abortion called for a physician's assistance, the Court recognized that the good physician is not just a mechanic of the human body whose services have no bearing on a person's moral choices, but one who does more than treat symptoms, one who ministers to the patient. See *id.,* at 153; see also *Griswold* v. *Connecticut,* 381 U.S., at 482 ("This law . . . operates directly on an intimate relation of husband and wife and their physician's role in one aspect of that relation"); see generally R. Cabot, Ether Day Address, Boston Medical and Surgical J. 287, 288 (1920). This idea of the physician as serving the whole person is a source of the high value traditionally placed on the medical relationship. Its value is surely as apparent here as in the abortion cases, for just as the decision about abortion is not directed to correcting some pathology, so the decision in which a dying patient seeks help is not so limited. The patients here sought not only an end to pain (which they might have had, although perhaps at the price of stupor) but an end to their short remaining lives with a dignity that they believed would be denied them by powerful pain medication, as well as by their consciousness of dependency and helplessness as they approached death. In that period when the end is imminent, they said, the decision to end life is closest to decisions that are generally accepted as proper instances of exercising autonomy over one's own body, instances recognized under the Constitution and the State's own law, instances in which the help of physicians is accepted as falling within the traditional norm.

Respondents argue that the State has in fact already recognized enough evolving examples of this tradition of patient care to demonstrate the strength of their claim. Washington, like other States, authorizes physicians to withdraw life sustaining medical treatment and artificially delivered food and water from patients who request it, even though such actions will hasten death. See Wash. Rev. Code §§70.122.110, 70.122.051 (1994); see generally Notes to Uniform Rights of the Terminally Ill Act, 9B U. L. A. 168-169 (Supp. 1997) (listing state statutes). The State permits physicians to alleviate anxiety and discomfort when withdrawing artificial life supporting devices by administering medication that will hasten death even further. And it generally permits physicians to administer medication to patients in terminal conditions when the primary intent is to alleviate pain, even when the medication is so powerful as to hasten death and the patient chooses to receive it with that understanding. See Wash. Rev. Code §70.122.010 (1994); see generally P. Rousseau, Terminal Sedation in the Care of Dying Patients, 156 Archives of Internal Medicine 1785 (1996); Truog, Berde, Mitchell, & Grier, Barbiturates in the Care of the Terminally Ill, 327 New Eng. J. Med. 1678 (1992).[15]

The argument supporting respondents' position thus progresses through three steps of increasing forcefulness. First, it emphasizes the decriminalization of suicide. Reliance on this fact is sanctioned under the standard that looks not only to the tradition retained, but to society's occasional choices to reject traditions of the legal past. See *Poe* v. *Ullman,* 367 U.S., at 542 (Harlan, J., dissenting). While the common law prohibited both suicide and aiding a suicide, with the prohibition on aiding largely justified by the primary prohibition on self inflicted death itself, see , *e.g.*, American Law Institute, Model Penal Code §210.5, Comment 1, pp. 92-93, and n. 7 (1980), the State's rejection of the traditional treatment of the one leaves the criminality of the other open to questioning that previously would not have been appropriate. The second step in the argument is to emphasize that the State's own act of decriminalization gives a freedom of choice much like the individual's option in recognized instances of bodily autonomy. One of these, abortion, is a legal right to choose in spite of the interest a State may legitimately invoke in discouraging the practice, just as suicide is now subject to choice, despite a state interest in discouraging it. The third step is to emphasize that respondents claim a right to assistance not on the basis of some broad principle that would be subject to exceptions if that continuing interest of the State's in discouraging suicide were to be recognized at all. Respondents base their claim on the traditional right to medical care and counsel, subject to the limiting conditions of informed, responsible choice when death is imminent, conditions that support a strong analogy to rights of care in other situations in which medical counsel and assistance have been available as a matter of course. There can be no stronger claim to a physician's assistance than at the time when death is imminent, a moral judgment implied by the State's own recognition of the legitimacy of medical procedures necessarily hastening the moment of impending death.

In my judgment, the importance of the individual interest here, as within that class of "certain interests" demanding careful scrutiny of the State's contrary claim, see *Poe, supra,* at 543, cannot be gainsaid. Whether that interest might in some circumstances, or at some time, be seen as "fundamental" to the degree entitled to prevail is not, however, a conclusion that I need draw here, for I am satisfied that the State's interests described in the following section are sufficiently serious to defeat the present claim that its law is arbitrary or purposeless.

The State has put forward several interests to justify the Washington law as applied to physicians treating terminally ill patients, even those competent to make responsible choices: protecting life generally, Brief for Petitioners 33, discouraging suicide even if knowing and voluntary, *id.*, at 37-38, and protecting terminally ill patients from involuntary suicide and euthanasia, both voluntary and nonvoluntary, *id.*, at 34-35.

It is not necessary to discuss the exact strengths of the first two claims of justification in the present circumstances, for the third is dispositive for me. That third justification is different from the first two, for it addresses specific features of respondents' claim, and it opposes that claim not with a moral judgment contrary to respondents', but with a recognized state interest in the protection of nonresponsible individuals and those who do not stand in relation either to death or to their physicians as do the patients whom respondents describe. The State claims interests in protecting patients from mistakenly and involuntarily deciding to end their lives, and in guarding against both voluntary and involuntary euthanasia. Leaving aside any difficulties in coming to a clear concept of imminent death, mistaken decisions may result from inadequate palliative care or a terminal prognosis that turns out to be error; coercion and abuse may stem from the large medical bills that family members cannot bear or unreimbursed hospitals decline to shoulder. Voluntary and involuntary euthanasia may result once doctors are authorized to prescribe lethal medication in the first instance, for they might find it pointless to distinguish between patients who administer their own fatal drugs and those who wish not to, and their compassion for those who suffer may obscure the distinction between those who ask for death and those who may be unable to request it. The argument is that a progression would occur, obscuring the line between the ill and the dying, and between the responsible and the unduly influenced, until ultimately doctors and perhaps others would abuse a limited freedom to aid suicides by yielding to the impulse to end another's suffering under conditions going beyond the narrow limits the respondents propose. The State thus argues, essentially, that respondents' claim is not as narrow as it sounds, simply because no recognition of the interest they assert could be limited to vindicating those interests and affecting no others. The State says that the claim, in practical effect, would entail consequences that the State could, without doubt, legitimately act to prevent.

The mere assertion that the terminally sick might be pressured into suicide decisions by close friends and family members would not alone be very telling. Of course that is possible, not only because the costs of care might be more than family members could bear but simply because they might naturally wish to see an end of suffering for someone they love. But one of the points of restricting any right of assistance to physicians, would be to condition the right on an exercise of judgment by someone qualified to assess the patient's responsible capacity and detect the influence of those outside the medical relationship.

The State, however, goes further, to argue that dependence on the vigilance of physicians will not be enough. First, the lines proposed here (particularly the requirement of a knowing and voluntary decision by the patient) would be more difficult to draw than the lines that have limited other recently recognized due process rights. Limiting a state from prosecuting use of artificial contraceptives by married couples posed no practical threat to the State's capacity to regulate contraceptives in other ways that were assumed at the time of *Poe* to be legitimate; the trimester measurements of *Roe* and the viability determination of *Casey* were easy to make with a real degree of certainty. But the knowing and responsible mind is harder to assess.[16] Second, this difficulty could become the greater by combining with another fact within the realm of plausibility, that physicians simply would not be assiduous to preserve the line. They have compassion, and those who would be willing to assist in suicide at all might be the most susceptible to the wishes of a patient, whether the patient were technically quite responsible or not. Physicians, and their hospitals, have their own financial incentives, too, in this new age of managed care. Whether acting from compassion or under some other influence, a physician who would provide a drug for a patient to administer might well go the further step of administering the drug himself; so, the barrier between assisted suicide and euthanasia could become porous, and the line between voluntary and involuntary euthanasia as well.[17] The case for the slippery slope is fairly made out here, not because recognizing one due process right would leave a court with no principled basis to avoid recognizing another, but because there is a plausible case that the right claimed would not be readily containable by reference to facts about the mind that are matters of difficult judgment, or by gatekeepers who are subject to temptation, noble or not.

Respondents propose an answer to all this, the answer of state regulation with teeth. Legislation proposed in several States, for example, would authorize physician assisted suicide but require two qualified physicians to confirm the patient's diagnosis, prognosis, and competence; and would mandate that the patient make repeated requests witnessed by at least two others over a specified time span; and would impose reporting requirements and criminal penalties for various acts of coercion. See App. to Brief for State Legislators as *Amici Curiae* 1a-2a.

But at least at this moment there are reasons for caution in predicting the effectiveness of the teeth proposed. Respondents' proposals, as it turns out, sound much like the guidelines now in place in the Netherlands, the only place where experience with physician assisted suicide and euthanasia has yielded empirical evidence about how such regulations might affect actual practice. Dutch physicians must engage in consultation before proceeding, and must decide whether the patient's decision is voluntary, well considered, and stable, whether the request to die is enduring and made more than once, and whether the patient's future will involve unacceptable suffering. See C. Gomez, Regulating Death 40-43 (1991). There is, however, a substantial dispute today about what the Dutch experience shows. Some commentators marshall evidence that the Dutch guidelines have in practice failed to protect patients from involuntary euthanasia and have been violated with impunity. See, *e.g.*, H. Hendin, Seduced By Death 75-84 (1997) (noting many cases in which decisions intended to end the life of a fully competent patient were made without a request from the patient and without consulting the patient); Keown, Euthanasia in the Netherlands: Sliding Down the Slippery Slope?, in Euthanasia Examined 261, 289 (J. Keown ed. 1995) (guidelines have "proved signally ineffectual; non voluntary euthanasia is now widely practiced and increasingly condoned in the Netherlands"); Gomez, *supra*, at 104-113. This evidence is contested. See, *e.g.*, R. Epstein, Mortal Peril 322 (1997) ("Dutch physicians are not euthanasia enthusiasts and they are slow to practice it in individual cases"); R. Posner, Aging and Old Age 242, and n. 23 (1995) (noting fear of "doctors' rushing patients to their death" in the Netherlands "has not been substantiated and does not appear realistic"); Van der Wal, Van Eijk, Leenen, & Spreeuwenberg, Euthanasia and Assisted Suicide, 2, Do Dutch Family Doctors Act Prudently?, 9 Family Practice 135 (1992) (finding no serious abuse in Dutch practice). The day may come when we can say with some assurance which side is right, but for now it is the substantiality of the factual disagreement, and the alternatives for resolving it, that matter. They are, for me, dispositive of the due process claim at this time.

I take it that the basic concept of judicial review with its possible displacement of legislative judgment bars any finding that a legislature has acted arbitrarily when the following conditions are met: there is a serious factual controversy over the feasibility of recognizing the claimed right without at the same time making it impossible for the State to engage in an undoubtedly legitimate exercise of power; facts necessary to resolve the controversy are not readily ascertainable through the judicial process; but they are more readily subject to discovery through legislative fact-finding and experimentation. It is assumed in this case, and must be, that a State's interest in protecting those unable to make responsible decisions and those who make no decisions at all entitles the State to bar aid to any but a knowing and responsible person intending suicide, and to prohibit euthanasia. How, and how far, a State should act in that interest are judgments for the State, but the legitimacy of its action to deny a physician the option to aid any but the knowing and responsible is beyond question.

The capacity of the State to protect the others if respondents were to prevail is, however, subject to some genuine question, underscored by the responsible disagreement over the basic facts of the Dutch experience. This factual controversy is not open to a judicial resolution with any substantial degree of assurance at this time. It is not, of course, that any controversy about the factual predicate of a due process claim disqualifies a court from resolving it. Courts can recognize captiousness, and most factual issues can be settled in a trial court. At this point, however, the factual issue at the heart of this case does not appear to be one of those. The principal enquiry at the moment is into the Dutch experience, and I question whether an independent front line investigation into the facts of a foreign country's legal administration can be soundly undertaken through American courtroom litigation. While an extensive literature on any subject can raise the hopes for judicial understanding, the literature on this subject is only nascent. Since there is little experience directly bearing on the issue, the most that can be said is that whichever way the Court might rule today, events could overtake its assumptions, as experimentation in some jurisdictions confirmed or discredited the concerns about progression from assisted suicide to euthanasia.

Legislatures, on the other hand, have superior opportunities to obtain the facts necessary for a judgment about the present controversy. Not only do they have more flexible mechanisms for fact-finding than the Judiciary, but their mechanisms include the power to experiment, moving forward and pulling back as facts emerge within their own jurisdictions. There is, indeed, good reason to suppose that in the absence of a judgment for respondents here, just such experimentation will be attempted in some of the States. See, *e.g.*, Ore. Rev. Stat. Ann. §§127.800 *et seq.* (Supp. 1996); App. to Brief for State Legislators as *Amici Curiae* 1a (listing proposed statutes).

I do not decide here what the significance might be of legislative foot dragging in ascertaining the facts going to the State's argument that the right in question could not be confined as claimed. Sometimes a court may be bound to act regardless of the institutional preferability of the political branches as forums for addressing constitutional claims. See, e.g., *Bolling* v. *Sharpe,* 347 U.S. 497 (1954). Now, it is enough to say that our examination of legislative reasonableness should consider the fact that the Legislature of the State of Washington is no more obviously at fault than this Court is in being uncertain about what would happen if respondents prevailed today. We therefore have a clear question about which institution, a legislature or a court, is relatively more competent to deal with an emerging issue as to which facts currently unknown could be dispositive. The answer has to be, for the reasons already stated, that the legislative process is to be preferred. There is a closely related further reason as well.

One must bear in mind that the nature of the right claimed, if recognized as one constitutionally required, would differ in no essential way from other constitutional rights guaranteed by enumeration or derived from some more definite textual source than "due process." An unenumerated right should not therefore be recognized, with the effect of displacing the legislative ordering of things, without the assurance that its recognition would prove as durable as the recognition of those other rights differently derived. To recognize a right of lesser promise would simply create a constitutional regime too uncertain to bring with it the expectation of finality that is one of this Court's central obligations in making constitutional decisions. See *Casey*, 505 U.S., at 864-869.

Legislatures, however, are not so constrained. The experimentation that should be out of the question in constitutional adjudication displacing legislative judgments is entirely proper, as well as highly desirable, when the legislative power addresses an emerging issue like assisted suicide. The Court should accordingly stay its hand to allow reasonable legislative consideration. While I do not decide for all time that respondents' claim should not be recognized, I acknowledge the legislative institutional competence as the better one to deal with that claim at this time.

NOTES

1. A nonprofit corporation known as Compassion in Dying was also a plaintiff and appellee below but is not a party in this Court.

2. As I will indicate in some detail below, I see the challenge to the statute not as facial but as applied, and I understand it to be in narrower terms than those accepted by the Court.

3. The doctors also rely on the Equal Protection Clause, but that source of law does essentially nothing in a case like this that the Due Process Clause cannot do on its own.

4. The status of the Harlan dissent in *Poe* v. *Ullman*, 367 U.S. 497 (1961), is shown by the Court's adoption of its result in *Griswold* v. *Connecticut*, 381 U.S. 479 (1965), and by the Court's acknowledgment of its status and adoption of its reasoning in *Planned Parenthood of Southeastern Pa.* v. *Casey*, 505 U.S. 833, 848-849 (1992). See also *Youngberg* v. *Romeo*, 457 U.S. 307, 320 (1982) (citing Justice Harlan's *Poe* dissent as authority for the requirement that this Court balance "the liberty of the individual" and "the demands of an organized society"); *Roberts* v. *United States Jaycees*, 468 U.S. 609, 619 (1984); *Moore* v. *East Cleveland*, 431 U.S. 494, 500-506, and n. 12 (1977) (plurality opinion) (opinion for four Justices treating Justice Harlan's *Poe* dissent as a central explication of the methodology of judicial review under the Due Process Clause).

5. Coke indicates that prohibitions against deprivations without "due pro-

cess of law" originated in an English statute that "rendered" Magna Carta's "law of the land" in such terms. See 2 E. Coke, Institutes 50 (1797); see also E. Corwin, Liberty Against Government 90-91 (1948).

6. The *Slaughter House Cases* are important, of course, for their holding that the Privileges or Immunities Clause was no source of any but a specific handful of substantive rights. *Slaughter House Cases*, 16 Wall., at 74-80. To a degree, then, that decision may have led the Court to look to the Due Process Clause as a source of substantive rights. In *Twining* v. *New Jersey*, 211 U.S. 78, 95-97 (1908), for example, the Court of the Lochner Era acknowledged the strength of the case against *Slaughter House*'s interpretation of the Privileges or Immunities Clause but reaffirmed that interpretation without questioning its own frequent reliance on the Due Process Clause as authorization for substantive judicial review. See also J. Ely, Democracy and Distrust 14-30 (1980) (arguing that the Privileges or Immunities Clause and not the Due Process Clause is the proper warrant for courts' substantive oversight of state legislation). But the courts' use of due process clauses for that purpose antedated the 1873 decision, as we have seen, and would in time be supported in the *Poe* dissent, as we shall see.

7. Judge Johnson of the New York Court of Appeals had made the point more obliquely a century earlier when he wrote that, "the form of this declaration of right, 'no person shall be deprived of life, liberty or property, without due process of law,' necessarily imports that the legislature cannot make the mere existence of the rights secured the occasion of depriving a person of any of them, even by the forms which belong to 'due process of law.' For if it does not necessarily import this, then the legislative power is absolute." And, "To provide for a trial to ascertain whether a man is in the enjoyment of [any] of these rights, and then, as a consequence of finding that he is in the enjoyment of it, to deprive him of it, is doing indirectly just what is forbidden to be done directly, and reduces the constitutional provision to a nullity." *Wynehamer* v. *People*, 13 N.Y. 378, 420 (1856).

8. We have made it plain, of course, that not every law that incidentally makes it somewhat harder to exercise a fundamental liberty must be justified by a compelling counter interest. See *Casey*, 505 U.S., at 872-876 (joint opinion of O'Connor, Kennedy, and Souter, JJ.); *Carey* v. *Population Services Int'l*, 431 U.S. 678, 685-686 (1977) ("[A]n individual's [constitutionally protected] liberty to make choices regarding contraception does not . . . automatically invalidate every state regulation in this area. The business of manufacturing and selling contraceptives may be regulated in ways that do not [even] infringe protected individual choices"). But a state law that creates a "substantial obstacle," *Casey*, *supra*, at 877, for the exercise of a fundamental liberty interest requires a commensurably substantial justification in order to place the legislation within the realm of the reasonable.

9. Justice Harlan thus recognized just what the Court today assumes, that by insisting on a threshold requirement that the interest (or, as the Court puts it, the right) be fundamental before anything more than rational basis justification is required, the Court ensures that not every case will require the "complex balancing" that heightened scrutiny entails. See *ante*, at 17-18.

10. Our cases have used various terms to refer to fundamental liberty inter-

ests, see, *e.g., Poe*, 367 U.S., at 545 (Harlan, J., dissenting) ("'basic liberty'") (quoting *Skinner* v. *Oklahoma ex rel. Williamson*, 316 U.S. 535, 541 (1942)); *Poe, supra*, at 543 (Harlan, J., dissenting) ("certain interests" must bring "particularly careful scrutiny"); *Casey*, 505 U.S., at 851 ("protected liberty"); *Cruzan* v. *Director, Mo. Dept. of Health*, 497 U.S. 261, 278 (1990) ("constitutionally protected liberty interest"); *Youngberg* v. *Romeo*, 457 U.S., at 315 ("liberty interests"), and at times we have also called such an interest a "right" even before balancing it against the government's interest, see, *e.g., Roe* v. *Wade*, 410 U.S. 113, 153-154 (1973); *Carey* v. *Population Services Int'l, supra*, at 686, 688, and n. 5; *Poe*, 367 U.S., at 541 ("rights 'which are . . . *fundamental*'") (quoting *Corfield* v. *Coryell*, 4 Wash. C.C. 371, 380 (CC ED Pa. 1825)). Precision in terminology, however, favors reserving the label "right" for instances in which the individual's liberty interest actually trumps the government's countervailing interests; only then does the individual have anything legally enforceable as against the state's attempt at regulation.

11. Thus, as the *Poe* dissent illustrates, the task of determining whether the concrete right claimed by an individual in a particular case falls within the ambit of a more generalized protected liberty requires explicit analysis when what the individual wants to do could arguably be characterized as belonging to different strands of our legal tradition requiring different degrees of constitutional scrutiny. See also Tribe & Dorf, Levels of Generality in the Definition of Rights, 57 U. Chi. L. Rev. 1057, 1091 (1990) (abortion might conceivably be assimilated either to the tradition regarding women's reproductive freedom in general, which places a substantial burden of justification on the State, or to the tradition regarding protection of fetuses, as embodied in laws criminalizing feticide by someone other than the mother, which generally requires only rationality on the part of the State). Selecting among such competing characterizations demands reasoned judgment about which broader principle, as exemplified in the concrete privileges and prohibitions embodied in our legal tradition, best fits the particular claim asserted in a particular case.

12. The dual dimensions of the strength and the fitness of the government's interest are succinctly captured in the so called "compelling interest test," under which regulations that substantially burden a constitutionally protected (or "fundamental") liberty may be sustained only if "narrowly tailored to serve a compelling state interest," *Reno* v. *Flores*, 507 U.S. 292, 302 (1993); see also, *e.g., Roe* v. *Wade*, 410 U.S., at 155; *Carey* v. *Population Services Int'l*, 431 U.S., at 686. How compelling the interest and how narrow the tailoring must be will depend, of course, not only on the substantiality of the individual's own liberty interest, but also on the extent of the burden placed upon it, see *Casey*, 505 U.S., at 871-874 (opinion of O'Connor, Kennedy, and Souter, JJ.); *Carey, supra*, at 686.

13. Washington and New York are among the minority of States to have criminalized attempted suicide, though neither State still does so. See Brief for Members of the New York and Washington State Legislatures as *Amicus Curiae* 15, n. 8 (listing state statutes). The common law governed New York as a colony and the New York Constitution of 1777 recognized the common law, N.Y. Const. of 1777, Art. XXXV, and the state legislature recognized common

law crimes by statute in 1788. See Act of Feb. 21, 1788, ch. 37, §2, 1788 N.Y. Laws 664 (codified at 2 N.Y. Laws 242) (Jones & Varick 1789). In 1828, New York changed the common law offense of assisting suicide from murder to manslaughter in the first degree. See 2 N.Y. Rev. Stat. pt. 4, ch. 1, tit. 2, art. 1, §7, p. 661 (1829). In 1881, New York adopted a new penal code making attempted suicide a crime punishable by two years in prison, a fine, or both, and retaining the criminal prohibition against assisting suicide as manslaughter in the first degree. Act of July 26, 1881, ch. 676, §§ 172-178, 1881 N.Y. Laws (3 Penal Code), pp. 42-43 (codified at 4 N.Y. Consolidated Laws, Penal Law §§2300 to 2306, pp. 2809-2810 (1909)). In 1919, New York repealed the statutory provision making attempted suicide a crime. See Act of May 5, 1919, ch. 414, §1,1919 N.Y. Laws 1193. The 1937 New York Report of the Law Revision Commission found that the history of the ban on assisting suicide was "traceable into the ancient common law when a suicide or *felo de se* was guilty of crime punishable by forfeiture of his goods and chattels." State of New York, Report of the Law Revision Commission for 1937, p. 830. The Report stated that since New York had removed "all stigma [of suicide] as a crime" and that "since liability as an accessory could no longer hinge upon the crime of a principal, it was necessary to define it as a substantive offense." *Id.*, at 831. In 1965, New York revised its penal law, providing that a "person is guilty of manslaughter in the second degree when . . . he intentionally causes or aids another person to commit suicide." Penal Law, ch. 1030, 1965 N.Y. Laws at 2387 (codified at N.Y. Penal Law §125.15(3) (McKinney 1975)).

Washington's first territorial legislature designated assisting another "in the commission of self murder" to be manslaughter, see Act of Apr. 28, 1854, §17, 1854 Wash. Laws 78, and re enacted the provision in 1869 and 1873, see Act of Dec. 2, 1869, §17, 1869 Wash. Laws 201; Act of Nov. 10, 1873, §19, 1873 Wash. Laws 184 (codified at Wash. Code §794 (1881)). In 1909, the state legislature enacted a law based on the 1881 New York law and a similar one enacted in Minnesota, see Marzen, O'Dowd, Crone, & Balch, 24 Duquesne L. Rev., at 206, making attempted suicide a crime punishable by two years in prison or a fine, and retaining the criminal prohibition against assisting suicide, designating it manslaughter. See Criminal Code, ch. 249, §§133-137, 1909 Wash. Laws, 11th Sess. 890, 929 (codified at Remington & Ballinger's Wash. Code §§2385-2389 (1910)). In 1975, the Washington Legislature repealed these provisions, see Wash. Crim. code, 1975, ch. 260, §9A.92.010 (213-217) 1975 Wash. Laws 817, 858, 866, and enacted the ban on assisting suicide at issue in this case, see Wash. Crim. code, 1975, ch. 260, §9A.36.060 1975 Wash. Laws 817, 836, codified at Rev. Wash. Code §§9A.36.060 (1977). The decriminalization of attempted suicide reflected the view that a person compelled to attempt it should not be punished if the attempt proved unsuccessful. See *Compassion in Dying* v. *Washington*, 850 F. Supp. 1454, 1464, n. 9 (WD Wash. 1994) (citing Legislative Council Judiciary Committee, Report on the Revised Washington Criminal Code 153 (Dec. 3, 1970).

14. Numerous States have enacted statutes prohibiting assisting a suicide. See, *e.g.*, Alaska Stat. Ann. §11.41.120(a)(2) (1996); Ariz. Rev. Stat. Ann. §13-1103(A)(3) (West Supp. 1996-1997); Ark. Code Ann. §5-10-104(a)(2) (1993);

Cal. Penal Code Ann. §401 (West 1988); Colo. Rev. Stat. §18-3-104(1)(b) (Supp. 1996); Conn. Gen. Stat. §53a 56(a)(2) (1997); Del. Code Ann. Tit. 11, §645 (1995); Fla. Stat. §782.08 (1991); Ga. Code Ann. §16-5-5(b) (1996); Haw. Rev. Stat. §707-702(1)(b) (1993); Ill. Comp. Stat., ch. 720, §5/12-31 (1993); Ind. Stat. Ann. §§35-42-1-2 to 35-42-1-2.5 (1994 and Supp. 1996); Iowa Code Ann. §707A.2 (West Supp. 1997); Kan. Stat. Ann. §21-3406 (1995); Ky. Rev. Stat. Ann. §216.302 (Michie 1994); La. Rev. Stat. Ann. §14:32.12 (West Supp. 1997); Me. Rev. Stat. Ann., Tit. 17-A, §204 (1983); Mich. Comp. Laws Ann. §752.1027 (West Supp. 1997-1998); Minn. Stat. §609.215 (1996); Miss. Code Ann. §97-3-49 (1994); Mo. Stat. §565.023.1(2) (1994); Mont. Code Ann. §45-5-105 (1995); Neb. Rev. Stat. §28-307 (1995); N. H. Rev. Stat. Ann. §630:4 (1996); N.J. Stat. Ann. §2C:11-6 (West 1995); N. M. Stat. Ann. §30-2-4 (1996); N.Y. Penal Law §120.30 (McKinney 1987); N. D. Cent. Code §12.1-16-04 (Supp. 1995); Okla. Stat. Tit. 21, §§813-815 (1983); Ore. Rev. Stat. §163.125(1)(b) (1991); Pa. Cons. Stat. Ann., Tit. 18 Purdon §2505 (1983); R. I. Gen. Laws §§11-60-1 through 11-60-5 (Supp. 1996); S. D. Codified Laws §22-16-37 (1988); Tenn. Code Ann. §39-13-216 (Supp. 1996); Tex. Penal Code Ann. §22.08 (1994); Wash. Rev. Code §9A.36.060 (1994); Wis. Stat. §940.12 (1993-1994). See also P. R. Law Ann., Tit. 33, § 4009 (1984).

15. Other States have enacted similar provisions, some categorically authorizing such pain treatment, see, *e.g.*, Ind. Code Ann. §35-42-1-2.5(a)(1) (Supp. 1996) (ban on assisted suicide does not apply to licensed health care provider who administers or dispenses medications or procedures to relieve pain or discomfort, even if such medications or procedures hasten death, unless provider intends to cause death); Iowa Code Ann. §707A.3.1 (West Supp. 1997) (same); Ky. Rev. Stat. Ann. §216.304 (Michie 1997) (same); Minn. Stat. Ann. §609.215(3) (West Supp. 1997) (same); Ohio Rev. Code Ann. §§2133.11(A)(6), 2133.12(E)(1) (1994); R. I. Gen. Laws §11-60-4 (Supp. 1996) (same); S. D. Codified Laws §22-16-37.1 (Supp. 1997); see Mich. Comp. Laws Ann. §752.1027(3) (West Supp. 1997); Tenn. Code Ann. §39-13-216(b)(2) (1996); others permit patients to sign health care directives in which they authorize pain treatment even if it hastens death. See, *e.g.*, Me. Rev. Stat. Ann., Tit. 18-A, §§5-804, 5-809 (1996); N. M. Stat. Ann. §§24-7A%4, 24-7A%9 (Supp. 1995); S. C. Code Ann. §62-5-504 (Supp. 1996); Va. Code Ann. §§54.1-2984, 4.1-2988 (1994).

16. While it is also more difficult to assess in cases involving limitations on life incidental to pain medication and the disconnection of artificial life support, there are reasons to justify a lesser concern with the punctilio of responsibility in these instances. The purpose of requesting and giving the medication is presumably not to cause death but to relieve the pain so that the State's interest in preserving life is not unequivocally implicated by the practice; and the importance of pain relief is so clear that there is less likelihood that relieving pain would run counter to what a responsible patient would choose, even with the consequences for life expectancy. As for ending artificial life support, the State again may see its interest in preserving life as weaker here than in the general case just because artificial life support preserves life when nature would not; and, because such life support is a frequently offensive bodily in-

trusion, there is a lesser reason to fear that a decision to remove it would not be the choice of one fully responsible. Where, however, a physician writes a prescription to equip a patient to end life, the prescription is written to serve an affirmative intent to die (even though the physician need not and probably does not characteristically have an intent that the patient die but only that the patient be equipped to make the decision). The patient's responsibility and competence are therefore crucial when the physician is presented with the request.

17. Again, the same can be said about life support and shortening life to kill pain, but the calculus may be viewed as different in these instances, as noted just above.

Supreme Court of the United States

WASHINGTON ET AL., PETITIONERS 96-110 v. HAROLD
GLUCKSBERG ET AL.
ON WRIT OF CERTIORARI TO THE UNITED STATES COURT OF APPEALS
FOR THE NINTH CIRCUIT
DENNIS C. VACCO, ATTORNEY GENERAL OF NEW YORK,
ET AL., PETITIONERS 95-1858 v. TIMOTHY E. QUILL
ET AL.
ON WRIT OF CERTIORARI TO THE UNITED STATES COURT OF
APPEALS FOR THE SECOND CIRCUIT
[JUNE 26, 1997]

Justice Ginsburg, concurring in the judgments.
I concur in the Court's judgments in these cases substantially for the reasons stated by Justice O'Connor in her concurring opinion.

Supreme Court of the United States

WASHINGTON ET AL., PETITIONERS 96-110 v. HAROLD
GLUCKSBERG ET AL.
ON WRIT OF CERTIORARI TO THE UNITED STATES COURT OF APPEALS

DENNIS C. VACCO, ATTORNEY GENERAL OF NEW YORK,
ET AL., PETITIONERS 95-1858 *v.* TIMOTHY E. QUILL
ET AL.

ON WRIT OF CERTIORARI TO THE UNITED STATES COURT OF
APPEALS FOR THE SECOND CIRCUIT

[JUNE 26, 1997]

Justice Breyer, concurring in the judgments.

I believe that Justice O'Connor's views, which I share, have greater legal significance than the Court's opinion suggests. I join her separate opinion, except insofar as it joins the majority. And I concur in the judgments. I shall briefly explain how I differ from the Court.

I agree with the Court in *Vacco* v. *Quill, ante,* that the articulated state interests justify the distinction drawn between physician assisted suicide and withdrawal of life support. I also agree with the Court that the critical question in both of the cases before us is whether "the 'liberty' specially protected by the Due Process Clause includes a right" of the sort that the respondents assert. *Washington* v. *Glucksberg, ante,* at 19. I do not agree, however, with the Court's formulation of that claimed "liberty" interest. The Court describes it as a "right to commit suicide with another's assistance." *Ante,* at 20. But I would not reject the respondents' claim without considering a different formulation, for which our legal tradition may provide greater support. That formulation would use words roughly like a "right to die with dignity." But irrespective of the exact words used, at its core would lie personal control over the manner of death, professional medical assistance, and the avoidance of unnecessary and severe physical suffering—combined.

As Justice Souter points out, *ante* at 13-16 (Souter, J., concurring in the judgment), Justice Harlan's dissenting opinion in *Poe* v. *Ullman,* 367 U.S. 497 (1961), offers some support for such a claim. In that opinion, Justice Harlan referred to the "liberty" that the Fourteenth Amendment protects as including "a freedom from all substantial arbitrary impositions and purposeless restraints" and also as recognizing that "*certain interests* require particularly careful scrutiny of the state needs asserted to justify their abridgment." *Id.,* at 543. The "certain interests" to which Justice Harlan referred may well be similar (perhaps identical) to the rights, liberties, or interests that the Court today, as in the past, regards as "fundamental." *Ante,* at 15; see also *Planned Parenthood of Southeastern Pa.* v. *Casey,* 505 U.S. 833 (1992); *Eisenstadt* v. *Baird,* 405 U.S. 438 (1972); *Griswold* v. *Connecticut,* 381 U.S. 479 (1965); *Rochin* v. *California,* 342 U.S. 165 (1952); *Skinner* v. *Oklahoma ex rel. Williamson,* 316 U.S. 535 (1942).

Justice Harlan concluded that marital privacy was such a "special interest." He found in the Constitution a right of "privacy of the home"—with the home, the bedroom, and "intimate details of the marital relation" at its heart—by examining the protection that the law had earlier provided for related, but not identical, interests described by such words as "privacy," "home," and "family." 367 U.S., at 548, 552; cf. *Casey, supra,* at 851. The respondents here essentially ask us to do the same. They argue that one can find a "right to die with dignity" by examining the protection the law has provided for related, but not identical, interests relating to personal dignity, medical treatment, and freedom from state inflicted pain. See *Ingraham* v. *Wright,* 430 U.S. 651 (1977); *Cruzan* v. *Director, Mo. Dept. of Health,* 497 U.S. 261 (1990); *Casey, supra.*

I do not believe, however, that this Court need or now should decide whether or a not such a right is "fundamental." That is because, in my view, the avoidance of severe physical pain (connected with death) would have to comprise an essential part of any successful claim and because, as Justice O'Connor points out, the laws before us do not *force* a dying person to undergo that kind of pain. *Ante,* at 2 (O'Connor, J., concurring). Rather, the laws of New York and of Washington do not prohibit doctors from providing patients with drugs sufficient to control pain despite the risk that those drugs themselves will kill. Cf. New York State Task Force on Life and the Law, When Death Is Sought: Assisted Suicide and Euthanasia in the Medical Context 163, n. 29 (May 1994). And under these circumstances the laws of New York and Washington would overcome any remaining significant interests and would be justified, regardless.

Medical technology, we are repeatedly told, makes the administration of pain relieving drugs sufficient, except for a very few individuals for whom the ineffectiveness of pain control medicines can mean, not pain, but the need for sedation which can end in a coma. Brief for National Hospice Organization 8; Brief for the American Medical Association (AMA) et al. as *Amici Curiae* 6; see also Byock, Consciously Walking the Fine Line: Thoughts on a Hospice Response to Assisted Suicide and Euthanasia, 9 J. Palliative Care 25, 26 (1993); New York State Task Force, at 44, and n. 37. We are also told that there are many instances in which patients do not receive the palliative care that, in principle, is available, *id.,* at 43-47; Brief for AMA as *Amici Curiae* 6; Brief for Choice in Dying, Inc., as *Amici Curiae* 20, but that is so for institutional reasons or inadequacies or obstacles, which would seem possible to overcome, and which do *not* include *a prohibitive set of laws. Ante,* at 2 (O'Connor, J., concurring); see also 2 House of Lords, Session 1993-1994 Report of Select Committee on Medical Ethics 113 (1994) (indicating that the number of palliative care centers in the United Kingdom, where physician assisted suicide is illegal, significantly exceeds that in the Netherlands, where such practices are legal).

This legal circumstance means that the state laws before us do not infringe directly upon the (assumed) central interest (what I have called the core of the interest in dying with dignity) as, by way of contrast, the state anticontraceptive laws at issue in *Poe* did interfere with the central interest there at stake —by bringing the State's police powers to bear upon the marital bedroom.

Were the legal circumstances different—for example, were state law to prevent the provision of palliative care, including the administration of drugs as needed to avoid pain at the end of life—then the law's impact upon serious and otherwise unavoidable physical pain (accompanying death) would be more directly at issue. And as Justice O'Connor suggests, the Court might have to revisit its conclusions in these cases.

APPENDIX D

Supreme Court of the United States

SYLLABUS

VACCO, ATTORNEY GENERAL OF NEW YORK, ET AL. *v.* QUILL
ET AL., 117 S.CT. 2293

ON WRIT OF CERTIORARI TO THE UNITED STATES COURT OF APPEALS
FOR THE SECOND CIRCUIT

No. 96-110

ARGUED JANUARY 8, 1997

DECIDED JUNE 26, 1997

In New York, as in most States, it is a crime to aid another to commit or attempt suicide, but patients may refuse even lifesaving medical treatment. Respondent New York physicians assert that, although it would be consistent with the standards of their medical practices to prescribe lethal medication for mentally competent, terminally ill patients who are suffering great pain and desire a doctor's help in taking their own lives, they are deterred from doing so by New York's assisted suicide ban. They, and three gravely ill patients who have since died, sued the State's Attorney General, claiming that the ban violates the Fourteenth Amendment's Equal Protection Clause. The Federal District Court disagreed, but the Second Circuit reversed, holding (1) that New York accords different treatment to those competent, terminally ill persons who wish to hasten their deaths by self administering prescribed drugs than it does to those who wish to do so by directing the removal of life support systems, and (2) that this supposed unequal treatment is not rationally related to any legitimate state interests.

Held: New York's prohibition on assisting suicide does not violate the Equal Protection Clause. Pp. 3-14.

(a) The Equal Protection Clause embodies a general rule that States must treat like cases alike but may treat unlike cases accordingly. *E.g., Plyler* v. *Doe,* 457 U.S. 202, 216. The New York statutes outlawing assisted suicide neither infringe fundamental rights nor involve suspect classifications, *e.g., Washington* v. *Glucksberg, ante,* at 14-24, and are therefore entitled to a strong presumption of validity, *Heller* v. *Doe,* 509 U.S. 312, 319. On their faces, neither the assisted suicide ban nor the law permitting patients to refuse medical treatment treats anyone differently from anyone else or draws any distinctions between persons. *Everyone,* regardless of physical condition, is entitled, if competent, to refuse unwanted lifesaving medical treatment; *no one* is permitted to assist a suicide. Generally, laws that apply evenhandedly to all unquestionably comply with equal protection. *E.g., New York City Transit Authority* v. *Beazer,* 440 U.S. 568, 587. This Court disagrees with the Second Circuit's submission that ending or refusing lifesaving medical treatment "is nothing more nor less than assisted suicide." The distinction between letting a patient die and making that patient die is important, logical, rational, and well established: It comports with fundamental legal principles of causation, see, *e.g., People* v. *Kevorkian,* 447 Mich. 436, 470-472, 527 N. W. 2d 714, 728, cert. denied, 514 U.S. 1083, and intent, see, *e.g., United States* v. *Bailey,* 444 U.S. 394, 403-406; has been recognized, at least implicitly, by this Court in *Cruzan* v. *Director, Mo. Dept. of Health,* 497 U.S. 261, 278-280; *id.,* at 287-288 (O'Connor, J., concurring); and has been widely recognized and endorsed in the medical profession, the state courts, and the overwhelming majority of state legislatures, which, like New York's, have permitted the former while prohibiting the latter. The Court therefore disagrees with respondents' claim that the distinction is "arbitrary" and "irrational." The line between the two acts may not always be clear, but certainty is not required, even were it possible. Logic and contemporary practice support New York's judgment that the two acts are different, and New York may therefore, consistent with the Constitution, treat them differently. Pp. 3-13.

(b) New York's reasons for recognizing and acting on the distinction between refusing treatment and assisting a suicide—including prohibiting intentional killing and preserving life; preventing suicide; maintaining physicians' role as their patients' healers; protecting vulnerable people from indifference, prejudice, and psychological and financial pressure to end their lives; and avoiding a possible slide towards euthanasia—are valid and important public interests that easily satisfy the constitutional requirement that a legislative classification bear a rational relation to some legitimate end. See *Glucksberg, ante.* Pp. 13-14.

80 F. 3d 716, reversed.

Rehnquist, C. J., delivered the opinion of the Court, in which O'Connor, Scalia, Kennedy, and Thomas, JJ., joined. O'Connor, J., filed a concurring opinion, in which Ginsburg and Breyer, JJ., joined in part. Stevens, J., Souter, J., Ginsburg, J., and Breyer, J., filed opinions concurring in the judgment.

Supreme Court of the United States

No. 95-1858

DENNIS C. VACCO, ATTORNEY GENERAL OF NEW YORK, ET AL., PETITIONERS *v.* TIMOTHY E. QUILL ET AL.

Chief Justice Rehnquist delivered the opinion of the Court.

In New York, as in most States, it is a crime to aid another to commit or attempt suicide,[1] but patients may refuse even lifesaving medical treatment.[2] The question presented by this case is whether New York's prohibition on assisting suicide therefore violates the Equal Protection Clause of the Fourteenth Amendment. We hold that it does not.

Petitioners are various New York public officials. Respondents Timothy E. Quill, Samuel C. Klagsbrun, and Howard A. Grossman are physicians who practice in New York. They assert that although it would be "consistent with the standards of [their] medical practice[s]" to prescribe lethal medication for "mentally competent, terminally ill patients" who are suffering great pain and desire a doctor's help in taking their own lives, they are deterred from doing so by New York's ban on assisting suicide. App. 25-26.[3] Respondents, and three gravely ill patients who have since died,[4] sued the State's Attorney General in the United States District Court. They urged that because New York permits a competent person to refuse life sustaining medical treatment, and because the refusal of such treatment is "essentially the same thing" as physician assisted suicide, New York's assisted suicide ban violates the Equal Protection Clause. *Quill* v. *Koppell*, 870 F. Supp. 78, 84-85 (SDNY 1994).

The District Court disagreed: "[I]t is hardly unreasonable or irrational for the State to recognize a difference between allowing nature to take its course, even in the most severe situations, and intentionally using an artificial death producing device." *Id.*, at 84. The court noted New York's "obvious legitimate interests in preserving life, and in protecting vulnerable persons," and concluded that "[u]nder the United States Constitution and the federal system it establishes, the resolution of this issue is left to the normal democratic processes within the State." *Id.*, at 84-85.

The Court of Appeals for the Second Circuit reversed. 80 F. 3d 716 (1996). The court determined that, despite the assisted suicide ban's apparent general applicability, "New York law does not treat equally all competent persons who are in the final stages of fatal illness and wish to hasten their deaths," because "those in the final stages of terminal illness who are on life support systems are allowed to hasten their deaths by directing the removal of such systems; but those who are similarly situated, except for the previous attachment of life sustaining equipment, are not allowed to hasten death by self administering prescribed drugs." *Id.*, at 727, 729. In the court's view, "[t]he ending of life by [the withdrawal of life support systems] is *nothing more nor less than assisted suicide.*" *Id.*, at 729 (emphasis added) (citation omitted). The Court of Appeals then examined whether this supposed unequal treatment was rationally related to any legitimate state interests,[5] and concluded that "to the extent that [New York's statutes] prohibit a physician from prescribing medications to be self administered by a mentally competent, terminally ill person in the final stages of his terminal illness, they are not rationally related to any legitimate state interest." *Id.*, at 731. We granted certiorari, 518 U.S. ____ (1996), and now reverse.

The Equal Protection Clause commands that no State shall "deny to any person within its jurisdiction the equal protection of the laws." This provision creates no substantive rights. *San Antonio Independent School Dist.* v. *Rodriguez*, 411 U.S. 1, 33 (1973); *id.*, at 59 (Stewart, J., concurring). Instead, it embodies a general rule that States must treat like cases alike but may treat unlike cases accordingly. *Plyler* v. *Doe*, 457 U.S. 202, 216 (1982) ("'[T]he Constitution does not require things which are different in fact or opinion to be treated in law as though they were the same'") (quoting *Tigner* v. *Texas*, 310 U.S. 141, 147 (1940)). If a legislative classification or distinction "neither burdens a fundamental right nor targets a suspect class, we will uphold [it] so long as it bears a rational relation to some legitimate end." *Romer* v. *Evans*, 517 U.S. ____, ____ (slip op., at 10) (1996).

New York's statutes outlawing assisting suicide affect and address matters of profound significance to all New Yorkers alike. They neither infringe fundamental rights nor involve suspect classifications. *Washington* v. *Glucksberg, ante,* at 15-24; see 80 F. 3d, at 726; *San Antonio School Dist.*, 411 U.S., at 28 ("The system of alleged discrimination and the class it defines have none of the traditional indicia of suspectness"); *id.*, at 33-35 (courts must look to the Constitution, not the "importance" of the asserted right, when deciding whether an asserted right is "fundamental"). These laws are therefore entitled to a "strong presumption of validity." *Heller* v. *Doe*, 509 U.S. 312, 319 (1993).

On their faces, neither New York's ban on assisting suicide nor its statutes permitting patients to refuse medical treatment treat anyone differently than anyone else or draw any distinctions between persons. *Everyone,* regardless of physical condition, is entitled, if competent, to refuse unwanted lifesaving medical treatment; *no one* is permitted to assist a suicide. Generally speaking, laws that apply evenhandedly to all "unquestionably comply" with the Equal Protection Clause. *New York City Transit Authority* v. *Beazer,* 440 U.S. 568, 587 (1979); see *Personnel Administrator of Mass.* v. *Feeney,* 442 U.S. 256, 271-273 (1979) ("[M]any [laws] affect certain groups unevenly, even though the law itself treats them no differently from all other members of the class described by the law").

The Court of Appeals, however, concluded that some terminally ill people —those who are on life support systems—are treated differently than those who are not, in that the former may "hasten death" by ending treatment, but the latter may not "hasten death" through physician assisted suicide. 80 F. 3d, at 729. This conclusion depends on the submission that ending or refusing lifesaving medical treatment "is nothing more nor less than assisted suicide." *Ibid.* Unlike the Court of Appeals, we think the distinction between assisting suicide and withdrawing life sustaining treatment, a distinction widely recognized and endorsed in the medical profession[6] and in our legal traditions, is both important and logical; it is certainly rational. See *Feeney, supra,* at 272 ("When the basic classification is rationally based, uneven effects upon particular groups within a class are ordinarily of no constitutional concern").

The distinction comports with fundamental legal principles of causation and intent. First, when a patient refuses life sustaining medical treatment, he dies from an underlying fatal disease or pathology; but if a patient ingests lethal medication prescribed by a physician, he is killed by that medication. See, *e.g., People* v. *Kevorkian*, 447 Mich. 436, 470-472, 527 N. W. 2d 714, 728 (1994), cert. denied, 514 U.S. 1083 (1995); *Matter of Conroy*, 98 N.J. 321, 355, 486 A. 2d 1209, 1226 (1985) (when feeding tube is removed, death "result[s] . . . from [the patient's] underlying medical condition"); *In re Colyer*, 99 Wash. 2d 114, 123, 660 P. 2d 738, 743 (1983) ("[D]eath which occurs after the removal of life sustaining systems is from natural causes"); American Medical Association, Council on Ethical and Judicial Affairs, Physician Assisted Suicide, 10 Issues in Law & Medicine 91, 92 (1994) ("When a life sustaining treatment is declined, the patient dies primarily because of an underlying disease").

Furthermore, a physician who withdraws, or honors a patient's refusal to begin, life sustaining medical treatment purposefully intends, or may so intend, only to respect his patient's wishes and "to cease doing useless and futile or degrading things to the patient when [the patient] no longer stands to benefit from them." Assisted Suicide in the United States, Hearing before the Subcommittee on the Constitution of the House Committee on the Judiciary, 104th Cong., 2d Sess., 368 (1996) (testimony of Dr. Leon R. Kass). The same is true when a doctor provides aggressive palliative care; in some cases, pain-killing drugs may hasten a patient's death, but the physician's purpose and intent is, or maybe, only to ease his patient's pain. A doctor who assists a suicide, however, "must, necessarily and indubitably, intend primarily that the patient be made dead." *Id.*, at 367. Similarly, a patient who commits suicide with a doctor's aid necessarily has the specific intent to end his or her own life, while a patient who refuses or discontinues treatment might not. See, *e.g., Matter of Conroy, supra*, at 351, 486 A. 2d, at 1224 (patients who refuse life sustaining treatment "may not harbor a specific intent to die" and may instead "fervently wish to live, but to do so free of unwanted medical technology, surgery, or drugs"); *Superintendent of Belchertown State School* v. *Saikewicz*, 373 Mass. 728, 743, n. 11, 370 N. E. 2d 417, 426, n. 11 (1977) ("[I]n refusing treatment the patient may not have the specific intent to die").

The law has long used actors' intent or purpose to distinguish between two acts that may have the same result. See, *e.g., United States* v. *Bailey*, 444 U.S. 394, 403-406 (1980) ("[T]he . . . common law of homicide often distinguishes . . . between a person who knows that another person will be killed as the result of his conduct and a person who acts with the specific purpose of taking another's life"); *Morissette* v. *United States*, 342 U.S. 246, 250 (1952) (distinctions based on intent are "universal and persistent in mature systems of law"); M. Hale, 1 Pleas of the Crown 412 (1847) ("If A., with an intent to prevent gangrene beginning in his hand doth without any advice cut off his hand, by which he dies, he is not thereby *felo de se* for tho it was a voluntary act, yet it was not with an intent to kill himself"). Put differently, the law distinguishes actions taken "because of" a given end from actions taken "in spite of" their unintended but foreseen consequences. *Feeney*, 442 U.S., at 279; *Compassion in Dying* v. *Washington*, 79 F. 3d 790, 858 (CA9 1996) (Kleinfeld, J., dissenting) ("When General Eisenhower ordered American soldiers onto the beaches of

Normandy, he knew that he was sending many American soldiers to certain death. . . . His purpose, though, was to . . . liberate Europe from the Nazis").

Given these general principles, it is not surprising that many courts, including New York courts, have carefully distinguished refusing life sustaining treatment from suicide. See, *e.g.*, *Fosmire* v. *Nicoleau*, 75 N.Y. 2d 218, 227, and n. 2, 551 N. E. 2d 77, 82, and n. 2 (1990) ("[M]erely declining medical . . . care is not considered a suicidal act").[7] In fact, the first state court decision explicitly to authorize withdrawing lifesaving treatment noted the "real distinction between the self infliction of deadly harm and a self determination against artificial life support." *In re Quinlan*, 70 N.J. 10, 43, 52, and n. 9, 355 A. 2d 647, 665, 670, and n. 9, cert. denied *sub nom. Garger* v. *New Jersey*, 429 U.S. 922 (1976). And recently, the Michigan Supreme Court also rejected the argument that the distinction "between acts that artificially sustain life and acts that artificially curtail life" is merely a "distinction without constitutional significance—a meaningless exercise in semantic gymnastics," insisting that "the *Cruzan* majority disagreed and so do we." *Kevorkian*, 447 Mich., at 471, 527 N. W. 2d, at 728.[8]

Similarly, the overwhelming majority of state legislatures have drawn a clear line between assisting suicide and withdrawing or permitting the refusal of unwanted lifesaving medical treatment by prohibiting the former and permitting the latter. *Glucksberg, ante,* at 4-6, 11-15. And "nearly all states expressly disapprove of suicide and assisted suicide either in statutes dealing with durable powers of attorney in health care situations, or in 'living will' statutes." *Kevorkian*, 447 Mich., at 478-479, and nn. 53-54, 527 N. W. 2d, at 731-732, and nn. 53-54.[9] Thus, even as the States move to protect and promote patients' dignity at the end of life, they remain opposed to physician assisted suicide.

New York is a case in point. The State enacted its current assisted suicide statutes in 1965.[10] Since then, New York has acted several times to protect patients' common law right to refuse treatment. Act of Aug. 7, 1987, ch. 818, §1, 1987 N.Y. Laws 3140 ("Do Not Resuscitate Orders") (codified as amended at N.Y. Pub. Health Law §§2960-2979 (McKinney 1994 and Supp. 1997)); Act of July 22, 1990, ch. 752, §2, 1990 N.Y. Laws 3547 ("Health Care Agents and Proxies") (codified as amended at N.Y. Pub. Health Law §§2980-2994 (McKinney 1994 and Supp. 1997)). In so doing, however, the State has neither endorsed a general right to "hasten death" nor approved physician assisted suicide. Quite the opposite: The State has reaffirmed the line between "killing" and "letting die." See N.Y. Pub. Health Law §2989(3) (McKinney 1994) ("This article is not intended to permit or promote suicide, assisted suicide, or euthanasia"); New York State Task Force on Life and the Law, Life Sustaining Treatment: Making Decisions and Appointing a Health Care Agent 36-42 (July 1987); Do Not Resuscitate Orders: The Proposed Legislation and Report of the New York State Task Force on Life and the Law 15 (Apr. 1986). More recently, the New York State Task Force on Life and the Law studied assisted suicide and euthanasia and, in 1994, unanimously recommended against legalization. When Death is Sought: Assisted Suicide and Euthanasia in the Medical Context vii (1994). In the Task Force's view, "allowing decisions to forego

life sustaining treatment and allowing assisted suicide or euthanasia have radically different consequences and meanings for public policy." *Id.*, at 146.

This Court has also recognized, at least implicitly, the distinction between letting a patient die and making that patient die. In *Cruzan* v. *Director, Mo. Dept. of Health*, 497 U.S. 261, 278 (1990), we concluded that "[t]he principle that a competent person has a constitutionally protected liberty interest in refusing unwanted medical treatment may be inferred from our prior decisions," and we assumed the existence of such a right for purposes of that case, *id.*, at 279. But our assumption of a right to refuse treatment was grounded not, as the Court of Appeals supposed, on the proposition that patients have a general and abstract "right to hasten death," 80 F. 3d, at 727-728, but on well established, traditional rights to bodily integrity and freedom from unwanted touching, *Cruzan*, 497 U.S., at 278-279; *id.*, at 287-288 (O'Connor, J., concurring). In fact, we observed that "the majority of States in this country have laws imposing criminal penalties on one who assists another to commit suicide." *Id.*, at 280. *Cruzan* therefore provides no support for the notion that refusing life sustaining medical treatment is "nothing more nor less than suicide."

For all these reasons, we disagree with respondents' claim that the distinction between refusing lifesaving medical treatment and assisted suicide is "arbitrary" and "irrational." Brief for Respondents 44.[11] Granted, in some cases, the line between the two may not be clear, but certainty is not required, even were it possible.[12] Logic and contemporary practice support New York's judgment that the two acts are different, and New York may therefore, consistent with the Constitution, treat them differently. By permitting everyone to refuse unwanted medical treatment while prohibiting anyone from assisting a suicide, New York law follows a longstanding and rational distinction.

New York's reasons for recognizing and acting on this distinction—including prohibiting intentional killing and preserving life; preventing suicide; maintaining physicians' role as their patients' healers; protecting vulnerable people from indifference, prejudice, and psychological and financial pressure to end their lives; and avoiding a possible slide towards euthanasia—are discussed in greater detail in our opinion in *Glucksberg, ante*. These valid and important public interests easily satisfy the constitutional requirement that a legislative classification bear a rational relation to some legitimate end.[13]

The judgment of the Court of Appeals is reversed.

It is so ordered.

NOTES

1. N.Y. Penal Law §125.15 (McKinney 1987) ("Manslaughter in the second degree") provides: "A person is guilty of manslaughter in the second degree when . . . (3) He intentionally causes or aids another person to commit suicide. Manslaughter in the second degree is a class C felony." Section 120.30 ("Promoting a suicide attempt") states: "A person is guilty of promoting a suicide attempt when he intentionally causes or aids another person to attempt suicide. Promoting a suicide attempt is a class E felony." See generally, *Washington* v. *Glucksberg*, _____ U.S. _____ (1997), *ante*, at 4-15.

2. "It is established under New York law that a competent person may refuse medical treatment, even if the withdrawal of such treatment will result in
death." *Quill* v. *Koppell,* 870 F. Supp. 78, 84 (SDNY 1994); see N.Y. Pub. Health
Law, Art. 29-B, §§2960-2979 (McKinney 1993 & Supp. 1997) ("Orders Not to
Resuscitate") (regulating right of "adult with capacity" to direct issuance of
orders not to resuscitate); *id.,* §§2980-2994 ("Health Care Agents and Proxies") (allowing appointment of agents "to make . . . health care decisions on
the principal's behalf," including decisions to refuse lifesaving treatment).

3. Declaration of Timothy E. Quill, M. D., App. 42-49; Declaration of
Samuel C. Klagsbrun, M. D., *id.,* at 68-74; Declaration of Howard A. Grossman,
M. D., *id.,* at 84-89; 80 F. 3d 716, 719 (CA2 1996).

4. These three patients stated that they had no chance of recovery, faced
the "prospect of progressive loss of bodily function and integrity and increasing pain and suffering," and desired medical assistance in ending their lives.
App. 25-26; Declaration of William A. Barth, *id.,* at 96-98; Declaration of
George A. Kingsley, *id.,* at 99-102; Declaration of Jane Doe, *id.,* at 105-109.

5. The court acknowledged that because New York's assisted suicide statutes "do not impinge on any fundamental rights [or] involve suspect classifications," they were subject only to rational basis judicial scrutiny. 80 F. 3d, at
726-727.

6. The American Medical Association emphasizes the "fundamental difference between refusing life sustaining treatment and demanding a life ending
treatment." American Medical Association, Council on Ethical and Judicial Affairs, Physician Assisted Suicide, 10 Issues in Law & Medicine 91, 93 (1994);
see also American Medical Association, Council on Ethical and Judicial Affairs,
Decisions Near the End of Life, 267 JAMA 2229, 2230-2231, 2233 (1992)
("The withdrawing or withholding of life sustaining treatment is not inherently
contrary to the principles of beneficence and nonmaleficence," but assisted
suicide "is contrary to the prohibition against using the tools of medicine to
cause a patient's death"); New York State Task Force on Life and the Law,
When Death is Sought: Assisted Suicide and Euthanasia in the Medical Context
108 (1994) ("[Professional organizations] consistently distinguish assisted suicide and euthanasia from the withdrawing or withholding of treatment, and
from the provision of palliative treatments or other medical care that risk fatal
side effects"); Brief for the American Medical Association et al. as *Amici Curiae*
18-25. Of course, as respondents' lawsuit demonstrates, there are differences
of opinion within the medical profession on this question. See New York Task
Force, When Death is Sought, *supra,* at 104-109.

7. Thus, the Second Circuit erred in reading New York law as creating a
"right to hasten death"; instead, the authorities cited by the court recognize a
right to refuse treatment, and nowhere equate the exercise of this right with
suicide. *Schloendorff* v. *Society of New York Hospital,* 211 N.Y. 125, 129-130, 105
N. E. 92, 93 (1914), which contains Justice Cardozo's famous statement that
"[e]very human being of adult years and sound mind has a right to determine
what shall be done with his own body," was simply an informed consent case.
See also *Rivers* v. *Katz,* 67 N.Y. 2d 485, 495, 495 N. E. 2d 337, 343 (1986) (right

to refuse antipsychotic medication is not absolute, and may be limited when "the patient presents a danger to himself"); *Matter of Storar*, 52 N.Y. 2d 363, 377, n. 6, 420 N. E. 2d 64, 71, n. 6, cert. denied, 454 U.S. 858 (1981).

8. Many courts have recognized this distinction. See, *e.g.*, *Kevorkian* v. Thompson, 947 F. Supp. 1152, 1178, and nn. 20-21 (ED Mich. 1997); *In re Fiori*, 543 Pa. 592, 602, 673 A. 2d 905, 910 (1996); *Singletary* v. *Costello*, 665 So. 2d 1099, 1106 (Fla. App. 1996); *Laurie* v. *Senecal*, 666 A. 2d 806, 808-809 (R. I. 1995); *State ex rel. Schuetzle* v. *Vogel*, 537 N. W. 2d 358, 360 (N. D. 1995); *Thor* v. *Superior Court*, 5 Cal. 4th 725, 741-742, 855 P. 2d 375, 385-386 (1993); *DeGrella* v. *Elston*, 858 S. W. 2d 698, 707 (Ky. 1993); *People* v. *Adams*, 216 Cal. App. 3d 1431, 1440, 265 Cal. Rptr. 568, 573-574 (1990); *Guardianship of Jane Doe*, 411 Mass. 512, 522-523, 583 N. E. 2d 1263, 1270, cert. denied *sub nom. Doe* v. *Gross*, 503 U.S. 950 (1992); *In re L. W.*, 167 Wis. 2d 53, 83, 482 N. W. 2d 60, 71 (1992); *In re Rosebush*, 195 Mich. App. 675, 681, n. 2, 491 N. W. 2d 633, 636, n. 2 (1992); *Donaldson* v. *Van de Kamp*, 2 Cal. App. 4th 1614, 1619-1625, 4 Cal. Rptr. 2d 59, 61-64 (1992); *In re Lawrance*, 579 N. E. 2d 32, 40, n. 4 (Ind. 1991); *McKay* v. *Bergstedt*, 106 Nev. 808, 822-823, 801 P. 2d 617, 626-627 (1990); *In re Browning*, 568 So. 2d 4, 14 (Fla. 1990); *McConnell* v. *Beverly Enterprises Connecticut, Inc.*, 209 Conn. 692, 710, 553 A. 2d 596, 605 (1989); *State* v. *McAfee*, 259 Ga. 579, 581, 385 S. E. 2d 651, 652 (1989); *In re Grant*, 109 Wash. 2d 545, 563, 747 P. 2d 445, 454-455 (1987); *In re Gardner*, 534 A. 2d 947, 955-956 (Me. 1987); *Matter of Farrell*, 108 N.J. 335, 349-350, 529 A. 2d 404, 411 (1987); *Rasmussen* v. *Fleming*, 154 Ariz. 207, 218, 741 P. 2d 674, 685 (1987); *Bouvia* v. *Superior Court*, 179 Cal. App. 3d 1127, 1144-1145, 225 Cal. Rptr. 297, 306 (1986); *Von Holden* v. *Chapman*, 87 App. Div. 2d 66, 70, 450 N.Y. S. 2d 623, 627 (1982); *Bartling* v. *Superior Court*, 163 Cal. App. 3d 186, 196-197, 209 Cal. Rptr. 220, 225-226 (1984); *Foody* v. *Manchester Memorial Hospital*, 40 Conn. Sup. 127, 137, 482 A. 2d 713, 720 (1984); *In re P. V. W.*, 424 So. 2d 1015, 1022 (La. 1982); *Leach* v. *Akron General Medical Center*, 68 Ohio Misc. 1, 10, 426 N. E. 2d 809, 815 (Ohio Comm. Pleas 1980); *In re Severns*, 425 A. 2d 156, 161 (Del. Ch. 1980); *Satz* v. *Perlmutter*, 362 So. 2d 160, 162-163 (Fla. App. 1978); *Application of the President and Directors of Georgetown College*, 331 F. 2d 1000, 1009 (CADC), cert. denied, 377 U.S. 978 (1964); *Brophy* v. *New England Sinai Hospital*, 398 Mass. 417, 439, 497 N. E. 2d 626, 638 (1986). The British House of Lords has also recognized the distinction. *Airedale N. H. S. Trust* v. *Bland*, 2 W. L. R. 316, 368 (1993).

9. See Ala. Code §22-8A—10 (1990); Alaska Stat. Ann. §§18.12.080(a), (f) (1996); Ariz. Rev. Stat. Ann. §36-3210 (Supp. 1996); Ark. Code Ann. §§20-13-905(a), (f), 20-17-210(a),(g) (1991 and Supp. 1995); Cal. Health & Safety Code Ann. §§7191.5(a), (g) (West Supp. 1997); Cal. Prob. Code Ann. §4723 (West. Supp. 1997); Colo. Rev. Stat. §§15-14-504(4), 15-18-112(1), 15-18.5-101(3), 15-18.6-108 (1987 and Supp. 1996); Conn. Gen. Stat. §19a—575 (Supp. 1996); Del. Code Ann., Tit. 16, §2512 (Supp. 1996); D. C. Code Ann. §§6-2430, 21-2212 (1995 and Supp. 1996); Fla. Stat. §§765.309(1), (2) (Supp. 1997); Ga. Code Ann. §§31-32-11(b), 31-36-2(b) (1996); Haw. Rev. Stat. §327D—13 (1996); Idaho Code §39-152 (Supp. 1996); Ill. Comp. Stat., ch.

755, §§35/9(f), 40/5, 40/50, 45/2-1 (1992); Ind. Code §§16-36-1-13, 16-36-4-19, 30-5-5-17 (1994 and Supp. 1996); Iowa Code §§144A.11.1-144A.11.6, 144B.12.2 (1989 and West Supp. 1997); Kan. Stat. Ann. §65-28,109 (1985); Ky. Rev. Stat. Ann. §311.638 (Baldwin Supp. 1992); La. Rev. Stat. Ann. 40: §§1299.58.10(A), (B) (West 1992); Me. Rev. Stat. Ann., Tit. 18-A, §§5-813(b), (c) (West Supp. 1996); Mass. Gen. Laws 201D, §12 (Supp. 1997); Md. Health Code Ann. §5-611(c) (1994); Mich. Comp. Laws Ann. §700.496(20) (West 1995); Minn. Stat. §§145B.14, 145C.14 (Supp. 1997); Miss. Code Ann. §§41-41-117(2),41-41-119(1) (Supp. 1992); Mo. Rev. Stat. §§459.015.3, 459.055(5) (1992); Mont. Code Ann. §§50-9-205(1), (7), 50-10-104(1), (6) (1995); Neb. Rev. Stat. §§20-412(1), (7), 30-3401(3) (1995); N. H. Rev. Stat. Ann. §§137-H:10, 137-H:13, 137 J:1 (1996); N.J. Stat. Ann. §§26:2H—54(d), (e), 26:2H—77 (West 1996); N. M. Stat. Ann. §§24-7A—13(B)(1), (C) (Supp. 1995); N.Y. Pub. Health Law §2989(3) (1993); Nev. Rev. Stat. §449.670(2) (1996); N. C. Gen. Stat. §§90-320(b), 90-321(f) (1993); N. D. Cent. Code §§23-06.4-01, 23-06.5-01 (1991); Ohio Rev. Code Ann. §2133.12(A), (D) (Supp. 1996); Okla. Stat. Ann., Tit. 63, §§3101.2(C),3101.12(A),(G) (1996); 20 Pa. Cons. Stat. §5402(b) (Supp. 1996); R. I. Gen. Laws §§23-4.10-9(a), (f), 23-4.11-10(a), (f) (1996); S. C. Code Ann. §§44-77-130, 44-78-50(A), (C), 62-5-504(O) (Supp. 1996); S. D. Codified Laws §§34-12D—14, 34-12D—20 (1994); Tenn. Code Ann. §§32-11-110(a), 39-13-216 (Supp. 1996); Tex. Health & Safety Code Ann. §§672.017, 672.020, 672.021 (1992); Utah Code Ann. §§75-2-1116,75-2-1118 (1993); Va. Code Ann. §54.1-2990 (1994); Vt. Stat. Ann., Tit. 18, §5260 (1987); V. I. Code Ann., Tit. 19, §§198(a), (g) (1995); Wash. Rev. Code §§70.122.070(1), 70.122.100 (Supp. 1997); W. Va. Code §§16-30-10, 16-30A—16(a), 16-30B—2(b), 16-30B—13, 16-30C—14 (1995); Wis. Stat. §§154.11(1), (6), 154.25(7), 155.70(7) (Supp. 1996); Wyo. Stat. §§3-5-211, 35-22-109, 35-22-208 (1994 & Supp. 1996). See also, 42 U.S.C. § 14402(b)(1), (2), (4) ("Assisted Suicide Funding Restriction Act of 1997").

10. It has always been a crime, either by statute or under the common law, to assist a suicide in New York. See Marzen, O'Dowd, Crone, & Balch, Suicide: A Constitutional Right?, 24 Duquesne L. Rev. 1, 205-210 (1985) (Appendix).

11. Respondents also argue that the State irrationally distinguishes between physician assisted suicide and "terminal sedation," a process respondents characterize as "induc[ing] barbiturate coma and then starv[ing] the person to death." Brief for Respondents 48-50; see 80 F. 3d, at 729. Petitioners insist, however, that "'[a]lthough proponents of physician assisted suicide and euthanasia contend that terminal sedation is covert physician assisted suicide or euthanasia, the concept of sedating pharmacotherapy is based on informed consent and the principle of double effect.'" Reply Brief for Petitioners 12 (quoting P. Rousseau, Terminal Sedation in the Care of Dying Patients, 156 Archives Internal Med. 1785, 1785-1786 (1996)). Just as a State may prohibit assisting suicide while permitting patients to refuse unwanted lifesaving treatment, it may permit palliative care related to that refusal, which may have the foreseen but unintended "double effect" of hastening the patient's death. See New York Task Force, When Death is Sought, *supra*, n. 6, at 163 ("It is widely

recognized that the provision of pain medication is ethically and professionally acceptable even when the treatment may hasten the patient's death, if the medication is intended to alleviate pain and severe discomfort, not to cause death").

12. We do not insist, as Justice Stevens suggests, *ante,* at 14-15 (concurring opinion), that "in all cases there will in fact be a significant difference between the intent of the physicians, the patients or the families [in withdrawal of treatment and physician assisted suicide cases]." See 6-7, *supra* ("[A] physician who withdraws, or honors a patient's refusal to begin, life sustaining medical treatment purposefully intends, *or may so intend,* only to respect his patient's wishes. . . . The same is true when a doctor provides aggressive palliative care; . . . the physician's purpose and intent is, *or may be,* only to ease his patient's pain") (emphasis added). In the absence of omniscience, however, the State is entitled to act on the reasonableness of the distinction.

13. Justice Stevens observes that our holding today "does not foreclose the possibility that some applications of the New York statute may impose an intolerable intrusion on the patient's freedom." *Ante,* at 16 (concurring opinion). This is true, but, as we observe in *Glucksberg, ante,* at 31-32, n. 24, a particular plaintiff hoping to show that New York's assisted suicide ban was unconstitutional in his particular case would need to present different and considerably stronger arguments than those advanced by respondents here.

Supreme Court of the United States

WASHINGTON ET AL., PETITIONERS 96-110 *v.* HAROLD
GLUCKSBERG ET AL.
On Writ of Certiorari to the United States Court of Appeals
for the Ninth Circuit
DENNIS C. VACCO, ATTORNEY GENERAL OF NEW YORK, ET
AL., PETITIONERS 95-1858 *v.* TIMOTHY E. QUILL ET AL.
On Writ of Certiorari to the United States Court of Appeals
for the Second Circuit
[JUNE 26, 1997]

Justice O'Connor, concurring.*
  Death will be different for each of us. For many, the last days will be spent in physical pain and perhaps the despair that accompanies physical deteriora-

tion and a loss of control of basic bodily and mental functions. Some will seek medication to alleviate that pain and other symptoms.

The Court frames the issue in this case as whether the Due Process Clause of the Constitution protects a "right to commit suicide which itself includes a right to assistance in doing so," *ante*, at 18, and concludes that our Nation's history, legal traditions, and practices do not support the existence of such a right. I join the Court's opinions because I agree that there is no generalized right to "commit suicide." But respondents urge us to address the narrower question whether a mentally competent person who is experiencing great suffering has a constitutionally cognizable interest in controlling the circumstances of his or her imminent death. I see no need to reach that question in the context of the facial challenges to the New York and Washington laws at issue here. See *ante*, at 18 ("The Washington statute at issue in this case prohibits 'aid[ing] another person to attempt suicide,' . . . and, thus, the question before us is whether the 'liberty' specially protected by the Due Process Clause includes a right to commit suicide which itself includes a right to assistance in doing so"). The parties and *amici* agree that in these States a patient who is suffering from a terminal illness and who is experiencing great pain has no legal barriers to obtaining medication, from qualified physicians, to alleviate that suffering, even to the point of causing unconsciousness and hastening death. See Wash. Rev. Code §70.122.010 (1994); Brief for Petitioners in No. 95-1858, p. 15, n. 9; Brief for Respondents in No. 95-1858, p. 15. In this light, even assuming that we would recognize such an interest, I agree that the State's interests in protecting those who are not truly competent or facing imminent death, or those whose decisions to hasten death would not truly be voluntary, are sufficiently weighty to justify a prohibition against physician assisted suicide. *Ante*, at 27-30; *post*, at 11 (Stevens, J., concurring in judgments); *post*, at 33-39 (Souter, J., concurring in judgment).

Every one of us at some point may be affected by our own or a family member's terminal illness. There is no reason to think the democratic process will not strike the proper balance between the interests of terminally ill, mentally competent individuals who would seek to end their suffering and the State's interests in protecting those who might seek to end life mistakenly or under pressure. As the Court recognizes, States are presently undertaking extensive and serious evaluation of physician-assisted suicide and other related issues. *Ante*, at 11, 12-13; see *post*, at 36-39 (Souter, J., concurring in judgment). In such circumstances, "the . . . challenging task of crafting appropriate procedures for safeguarding . . . liberty interests is entrusted to the 'laboratory' of the States . . . in the first instance." *Cruzan* v. *Director, Mo. Dept. of Health,* 497 U.S. 261, 292 (1990) (O'Connor, J., concurring) (citing *New State Ice Co.* v. *Liebmann,* 285 U.S. 262, 311 (1932)).

In sum, there is no need to address the question whether suffering patients have a constitutionally cognizable interest in obtaining relief from the suffering that they may experience in the last days of their lives. There is no dispute that dying patients in Washington and New York can obtain palliative care, even when doing so would hasten their deaths. The difficulty in defining terminal illness and the risk that a dying patient's request for assistance in ending his or her life might not be truly voluntary justifies the prohibitions on assisted suicide we uphold here.

NOTES

* Justice Ginsburg concurs in the Court's judgments substantially for the reasons stated in this opinion. Justice Breyer joins this opinion except insofar as it joins the opinions of the Court.

Supreme Court of the United States

WASHINGTON ET AL., PETITIONERS 96-110 *v.* HAROLD GLUCKSBERG ET AL.

ON WRIT OF CERTIORARI TO THE UNITED STATES COURT OF APPEALS FOR THE NINTH CIRCUIT

DENNIS C. VACCO, ATTORNEY GENERAL OF NEW YORK, ET AL., PETITIONERS 95-1858 *v.* TIMOTHY E. QUILL ET AL.

ON WRIT OF CERTIORARI TO THE UNITED STATES COURT OF APPEALS FOR THE SECOND CIRCUIT

[JUNE 26, 1997]

Justice Stevens, concurring in the judgments.

The Court ends its opinion with the important observation that our holding today is fully consistent with a continuation of the vigorous debate about the "morality, legality, and practicality of physician assisted suicide" in a democratic society. *Ante,* at 32. I write separately to make it clear that there is also room for further debate about the limits that the Constitution places on the power of the States to punish the practice.

The morality, legality, and practicality of capital punishment have been the subject of debate for many years. In 1976, this Court upheld the constitutionality of the practice in cases coming to us from Georgia,[1] Florida,[2] and Texas.[3] In those cases we concluded that a State does have the power to place a lesser value on some lives than on others; there is no absolute requirement that a State treat all human life as having an equal right to preservation. Because the state legislatures had sufficiently narrowed the category of lives that the State could terminate, and had enacted special procedures to ensure that the defendant belonged in that limited category, we concluded that the statutes were not unconstitutional on their face. In later cases coming to us from each of those States, however, we found that some applications of the statutes were unconstitutional.[4]

Today, the Court decides that Washington's statute prohibiting assisted suicide is not invalid "on its face," that is to say, in all or most cases in which it might be applied.[5] That holding, however, does not foreclose the possibility that some applications of the statute might well be invalid.

As originally filed, this case presented a challenge to the Washington statute on its face and as it applied to three terminally ill, mentally competent patients and to four physicians who treat terminally ill patients. After the District Court issued its opinion holding that the statute placed an undue burden on the right to commit physician assisted suicide, see *Compassion in Dying* v. *Washington*, 850 F. Supp. 1454, 1462, 1465 (WD Wash. 1994), the three patients died. Although the Court of Appeals considered the constitutionality of the statute-as applied to the prescription of life ending medication for use by terminally ill, competent adult patients who wish to hasten their deaths," *Compassion in Dying* v. *Washington*, 79 F. 3d 790, 798 (CA9 1996), the court did not have before it any individual plaintiff seeking to hasten her death or any doctor who was threatened with prosecution for assisting in the suicide of a particular patient; its analysis and eventual holding that the statute was unconstitutional was not limited to a particular set of plaintiffs before it.

The appropriate standard to be applied in cases making facial challenges to state statutes has been the subject of debate within this Court. See *Janklow* v. *Planned Parenthood, Sioux Falls Clinic*, 517 U.S. _____ (1996). Upholding the validity of the federal Bail Reform Act of 1984, the Court stated in *United States* v. *Salerno*, 481 U.S. 739 (1987), that a "facial challenge to a legislative Act is, of course, the most difficult challenge to mount successfully, since the challenger must establish that no set of circumstances exists under which the Act would be valid." *Id.*, at 745.[6] I do not believe the Court has ever actually applied such a strict standard,[7] even in *Salerno* itself, and the Court does not appear to apply *Salerno* here. Nevertheless, the Court does conceive of respondents' claim as a facial challenge—addressing not the application of the statute to a particular set of plaintiffs before it, but the constitutionality of the statute's categorical prohibition against "aid[ing] another person to attempt suicide." *Ante*, at 18 (internal quotation marks omitted) (citing Wash. Rev. Code §9A.36.060(1) (1994)). Accordingly, the Court requires the plaintiffs to show that the interest in liberty protected by the Fourteenth Amendment "includes a right to commit suicide which itself includes a right to assistance in doing so." *Ante*, at 18.

History and tradition provide ample support for refusing to recognize an open ended constitutional right to commit suicide. Much more than the State's paternalistic interest in protecting the individual from the irrevocable consequences of an ill-advised decision motivated by temporary concerns is at stake. There is truth in John Donne's observation that "No man is an island."[8] The State has an interest in preserving and fostering the benefits that every human being may provide to the community—a community that thrives on the exchange of ideas, expressions of affection, shared memories and humorous incidents as well as on the material contributions that its members create and support. The value to others of a person's life is far too precious to allow the individual to claim a constitutional entitlement to complete autonomy in making a decision to end that life. Thus, I fully agree with the Court that the "liberty" protected by the Due Process Clause does not include a categorical "right to commit suicide which itself includes a right to assistance in doing so." *Ante,* at 18.

But just as our conclusion that capital punishment is not always unconstitutional did not preclude later decisions holding that it is sometimes impermissibly cruel, so is it equally clear that a decision upholding a general statutory prohibition of assisted suicide does not mean that every possible application of the statute would be valid. A State, like Washington, that has authorized the death penalty and thereby has concluded that the sanctity of human life does not require that it always be preserved, must acknowledge that there are situations in which an interest in hastening death is legitimate. Indeed, not only is that interest sometimes legitimate, I am also convinced that there are times when it is entitled to constitutional protection.

In *Cruzan v. Director, Mo. Dept. of Health,* 497 U.S. 261 (1990), the Court assumed that the interest in liberty protected by the Fourteenth Amendment encompassed the right of a terminally ill patient to direct the withdrawal of life sustaining treatment. As the Court correctly observes today, that assumption "was not simply deduced from abstract concepts of personal autonomy." *Ante,* at 21. Instead, it was supported by the common law tradition protecting the individual's general right to refuse unwanted medical treatment. *Ibid.* We have recognized, however, that this common law right to refuse treatment is neither absolute nor always sufficiently weighty to overcome valid countervailing state interests. As Justice Brennan pointed out in his *Cruzan* dissent, we have upheld legislation imposing punishment on persons refusing to be vaccinated, 497 U.S., at 312, n. 12, citing *Jacobson v. Massachusetts,* 197 U.S. 11, 26-27 (1905), and as Justice Scalia pointed out in his concurrence, the State ordinarily has the right to interfere with an attempt to commit suicide by, for example, forcibly placing a bandage on a self inflicted wound to stop the flow of blood. 497 U.S., at 298. In most cases, the individual's constitutionally protected interest in his or her own physical autonomy, including the right to refuse unwanted medical treatment, will give way to the State's interest in preserving human life.

Cruzan, however, was not the normal case. Given the irreversible nature of her illness and the progressive character of her suffering,[9] Nancy Cruzan's interest in refusing medical care was incidental to her more basic interest in controlling the manner and timing of her death. In finding that her best interests would be served by cutting off the nourishment that kept her alive, the trial court did more than simply vindicate Cruzan's interest in refusing medical treatment; the court, in essence, authorized affirmative conduct that would hasten her death. When this Court reviewed the case and upheld Missouri's requirement that there be clear and convincing evidence establishing Nancy Cruzan's intent to have life sustaining nourishment withdrawn, it made two important assumptions: (1) that there was a "liberty interest" in refusing unwanted treatment protected by the Due Process Clause; and (2) that this liberty interest did not "end the inquiry" because it might be outweighed by relevant state interests. *Id.*, at 279. I agree with both of those assumptions, but I insist that the source of Nancy Cruzan's right to refuse treatment was not just a common law rule. Rather, this right is an aspect of a far broader and more basic concept of freedom that is even older than the common law.[10] This freedom embraces, not merely a person's right to refuse a particular kind of unwanted treatment, but also her interest in dignity, and in determining the character of the memories that will survive long after her death.[11] In recognizing that the State's interests did not outweigh Nancy Cruzan's liberty interest in refusing medical treatment, *Cruzan* rested not simply on the common law right to refuse medical treatment, but—at least implicitly—on the even more fundamental right to make this "deeply personal decision," 497 U.S., at 289 (O'Connor, J., concurring).

Thus, the common law right to protection from battery, which included the right to refuse medical treatment in most circumstances, did not mark "the outer limits of the substantive sphere of liberty" that supported the Cruzan family's decision to hasten Nancy's death. *Planned Parenthood of Southeastern Pa. v. Casey*, 505 U.S. 833, 848 (1992). Those limits have never been precisely defined. They are generally identified by the importance and character of the decision confronted by the individual, *Whalen v. Roe*, 429 U.S. 589, 599-600, n. 26 (1977). Whatever the outer limits of the concept may be, it definitely includes protection for matters "central to personal dignity and autonomy." *Casey*, 505 U.S., at 851. It includes, "the individual's right to make certain unusually important decisions that will affect his own, or his family's, destiny. The Court has referred to such decisions as implicating 'basic values,' as being 'fundamental,' and as being dignified by history and tradition. The character of the Court's language in these cases brings to mind the origins of the American heritage of freedom—the abiding interest in individual liberty that makes certain state intrusions on the citizen's right to decide how he will live his own life intolerable." *Fitzgerald v. Porter Memorial Hospital*, 523 F. 2d 716, 719-720 (CA7 1975) (footnotes omitted), cert. denied, 425 U.S. 916 (1976).

The *Cruzan* case demonstrated that some state intrusions on the right to decide how death will be encountered are also intolerable. The now deceased plaintiffs in this action may in fact have had a liberty interest even stronger than Nancy Cruzan's because, not only were they terminally ill, they were suffering constant and severe pain. Avoiding intolerable pain and the indignity of living one's final days incapacitated and in agony is certainly "[a]t the heart of [the] liberty . . . to define one's own concept of existence, of meaning, of the universe, and of the mystery of human life." *Casey*, 505 U.S., at 851.

While I agree with the Court that *Cruzan* does not decide the issue presented by these cases, *Cruzan* did give recognition, not just to vague, unbridled notions of autonomy, but to the more specific interest in making decisions about how to confront an imminent death. Although there is no absolute right to physician assisted suicide, *Cruzan* makes it clear that some individuals who no longer have the option of deciding whether to live or to die because they are already on the threshold of death have a constitutionally protected interest that may outweigh the State's interest in preserving life at all costs. The liberty interest at stake in a case like this differs from, and is stronger than, both the common law right to refuse medical treatment and the unbridled interest in deciding whether to live or die. It is an interest in deciding how, rather than whether, a critical threshold shall be crossed.

The state interests supporting a general rule banning the practice of physician assisted suicide do not have the same force in all cases. First and foremost of these interests is the "'unqualified interest in the preservation of human life,'" *ante,* at 24, (quoting *Cruzan,* 497 U.S., at 282,) which is equated with "'the sanctity of life,'" *ante,* at 25, (quoting the American Law Institute, Model Penal Code §210.5, Comment 5, p. 100 (Official Draft and Revised Comments 1980)). That interest not only justifies—it commands—maximum protection of every individual's interest in remaining alive, which in turn commands the same protection for decisions about whether to commence or to terminate life support systems or to administer pain medication that may hasten death. Properly viewed, however, this interest is not a collective interest that should always outweigh the interests of a person who because of pain, incapacity, or sedation finds her life intolerable, but rather, an aspect of individual freedom.

Many terminally ill people find their lives meaningful even if filled with pain or dependence on others. Some find value in living through suffering; some have an abiding desire to witness particular events in their families' lives; many believe it a sin to hasten death. Individuals of different religious faiths make different judgments and choices about whether to live on under such circumstances. There are those who will want to continue aggressive treatment; those who would prefer terminal sedation; and those who will seek withdrawal from life support systems and death by gradual starvation and dehydration. Although as a general matter the State's interest in the contributions each person may make to society outweighs the person's interest in ending her life, this interest does not have the same force for a terminally ill patient faced not with the choice of whether to live, only of how to die. Allowing the individual, rather than the State, to make judgments "'about the "quality" of life that a particular individual may enjoy.'" *ante,* at 25 (quoting *Cruzan,* 497 U.S., at 282), does not mean that the lives of terminally ill, disabled people have less value than the lives of those who are healthy, see *ante,* at 28. Rather, it gives proper recognition to the individual's interest in choosing a final chapter that accords with her life story, rather than one that demeans her values and poisons memories of her. See Brief for Bioethicists as *Amici Curiae* 11; see also R. Dworkin, Life's Dominion 213 (1993) ("Whether it is in someone's best interests that his life end in one way rather than another depends on so much else that is special about him—about the shape and character of his life and his own sense of his integrity and critical interests—that no uniform collective decision can possibly hope to serve everyone even decently").

Similarly, the State's legitimate interests in preventing suicide, protecting the vulnerable from coercion and abuse, and preventing euthanasia are less significant in this context. I agree that the State has a compelling interest in preventing persons from committing suicide because of depression, or coercion by third parties. But the State's legitimate interest in preventing abuse does not apply to an individual who is not victimized by abuse, who is not suffering from depression, and who makes a rational and voluntary decision to seek assistance in dying. Although, as the New York Task Force report discusses, diagnosing depression and other mental illness is not always easy, mental health workers and other professionals expert in working with dying patients can help patients cope with depression and pain, and help patients assess their options. See Brief for Washington State Psychological Association et al. as *Amici Curiae* 8-10.

Relatedly, the State and *amici* express the concern that patients whose physical pain is inadequately treated will be more likely to request assisted suicide. Encouraging the development and ensuring the availability of adequate pain treatment is of utmost importance; palliative care, however, cannot alleviate all pain and suffering. See Orentlicher, Legalization of Physician Assisted Suicide: A Very Modest Revolution, 38 Boston College L. Rev. (Galley, p. 8) (1997) ("Greater use of palliative care would reduce the demand for assisted suicide, but it will not eliminate [it]"); see also Brief for Coalition of Hospice Professionals as *Amici Curiae* 8 (citing studies showing that "[a]s death becomes more imminent, pain and suffering become progressively more difficult to treat"). An individual adequately informed of the care alternatives thus might make a rational choice for assisted suicide. For such an individual, the State's interest in preventing potential abuse and mistake is only minimally implicated.

The final major interest asserted by the State is its interest in preserving the traditional integrity of the medical profession. The fear is that a rule permitting physicians to assist in suicide is inconsistent with the perception that they serve their patients solely as healers. But for some patients, it would be a physician's refusal to dispense medication to ease their suffering and make their death tolerable and dignified that would be inconsistent with the healing role See Block & Billings, Patient Request to Hasten Death, 154 Archives Internal Med. 2039, 2045 (1994) (A doctor's refusal to hasten death "may be experienced by the [dying] patient as an abandonment, a rejection, or an expression of inappropriate paternalistic authority"). For doctors who have long standing relationships with their patients, who have given their patients advice on alternative treatments, who are attentive to their patient's individualized needs, and who are knowledgeable about pain symptom management and palliative care options, see Quill, Death and Dignity, A Case of Individualized Decision Making, 324 New England J. of Med. 691-694 (1991), heeding a patient's desire to assist in her suicide would not serve to harm the physician patient relationship. Furthermore, because physicians are already involved in making decisions that hasten the death of terminally ill patients—through termination of life support, withholding of medical treatment, and terminal sedation—there is in fact significant tension between the traditional view of the physician's role and the actual practice in a growing number of cases.[12]

As the New York State Task Force on Life and the Law recognized, a State's prohibition of assisted suicide is justified by the fact that the "'ideal'" case in which "patients would be screened for depression and offered treatment, effective pain medication would be available, and all patients would have a supportive committed family and doctor" is not the usual case. New York State Task Force on Life and the Law, When Death Is Sought: Assisted Suicide and

Euthanasia in the Medical Context 120 (May 1994). Although, as the Court concludes today, these *potential* harms are sufficient to support the State's general public policy against assisted suicide, they will not always outweigh the individual liberty interest of a particular patient. Unlike the Court of Appeals, I would not say as a categorical matter that these state interests are invalid as to the entire class of terminally ill, mentally competent patients. I do not, however, foreclose the possibility that an individual plaintiff seeking to hasten her death, or a doctor whose assistance was sought, could prevail in a more particularized challenge. Future cases will determine whether such a challenge may succeed.

In New York, a doctor must respect a competent person's decision to refuse or to discontinue medical treatment even though death will thereby ensue, but the same doctor would be guilty of a felony if she provided her patient assistance in committing suicide.[13] Today we hold that the Equal Protection Clause is not violated by the resulting disparate treatment of two classes of terminally ill people who may have the same interest in hastening death. I agree that the distinction between permitting death to ensue from an underlying fatal disease and causing it to occur by the administration of medication or other means provides a constitutionally sufficient basis for the State's classification.[14] Unlike the Court, however, see *Vacco, ante,* at 6-7, I am not persuaded that in all cases there will in fact be a significant difference between the intent of the physicians, the patients or the families in the two situations.

There may be little distinction between the intent of a terminally ill patient who decides to remove her life support and one who seeks the assistance of a doctor in ending her life; in both situations, the patient is seeking to hasten a certain, impending death. The doctor's intent might also be the same in prescribing lethal medication as it is in terminating life support. A doctor who fails to administer medical treatment to one who is dying from a disease could be doing so with an intent to harm or kill that patient. Conversely, a doctor who prescribes lethal medication does not necessarily intend the patient's death—rather that doctor may seek simply to ease the patient's suffering and to comply with her wishes. The illusory character of any differences in intent or causation is confirmed by the fact that the American Medical Association unequivocally endorses the practice of terminal sedation—the administration of sufficient dosages of pain killing medication to terminally ill patients to protect them from excruciating pain even when it is clear that the time of death will be advanced. The purpose of terminal sedation is to ease the suffering of the patient and comply with her wishes, and the actual cause of death is the administration of heavy doses of lethal sedatives. This same intent and causation may exist when a doctor complies with a patient's request for lethal medication to hasten her death.[15]

Thus, although the differences the majority notes in causation and intent between terminating life support and assisting in suicide support the Court's rejection of the respondents' facial challenge, these distinctions may be inapplicable to particular terminally ill patients and their doctors. Our holding today in *Vacco* v. *Quill* that the Equal Protection Clause is not violated by New York's classification, just like our holding in *Washington* v. *Glucksberg* that the

Washington statute is not invalid on its face, does not foreclose the possibility that some applications of the New York statute may impose an intolerable intrusion on the patient's freedom.

There remains room for vigorous debate about the outcome of particular cases that are not necessarily resolved by the opinions announced today. How such cases may be decided will depend on their specific facts. In my judgment, however, it is clear that the so called "unqualified interest in the preservation of human life," *Cruzan,* 497 U.S., at 282, *Glucksberg, ante,* at 24, is not itself sufficient to outweigh the interest in liberty that may justify the only possible means of preserving a dying patient's dignity and alleviating her intolerable suffering.

NOTES

1. *Gregg* v. *Georgia,* 428 U.S. 153 (1976).

2. *Proffitt* v. *Florida,* 428 U.S. 242 (1976).

3. *Jurek* v. *Texas,* 428 U.S. 262 (1976).

4. See, *e.g., Godfrey* v. *Georgia,* 446 U.S. 420 (1980); *Enmund* v. *Florida,* 458 U.S. 782 (1982); *Penry* v. *Lynaugh,* 492 U.S. 302 (1989).

5. See *ante,* at 3, n. 5.

6. If the Court had actually applied the *Salerno* standard in this action, it would have taken only a few paragraphs to identify situations in which the Washington statute could be validly enforced. In *Salerno* itself, the Court would have needed only to look at whether the statute could be constitutionally applied to the arrestees before it; any further analysis would have been superfluous. See Dorf, Facial Challenges to State and Federal Statutes, 46 Stan. L. Rev. 235, 239-240 (1994) (arguing that if the *Salerno* standard were taken literally, a litigant could not succeed in her facial challenge unless she also succeeded in her as applied challenge).

7. In other cases and in other contexts, we have imposed a significantly lesser burden on the challenger. The most lenient standard that we have applied requires the challenger to establish that the invalid applications of a statute "must not only be real, but substantial as well, judged in relation to the statute's plainly legitimate sweep." *Broadrick* v. *Oklahoma,* 413 U.S. 601, 615 (1973). As the Court's opinion demonstrates, Washington's statute prohibiting assisted suicide has a "plainly legitimate sweep." While that demonstration provides a sufficient justification for rejecting respondents' facial challenge, it does not mean that every application of the statute should or will be upheld.

8. "Who casts not up his eye to the sun when it rises? but who takes off his eye from a comet when that breaks out? Who bends not his ear to any bell which upon any occasion rings? but who can remove it from that bell which is passing a piece of himself out of this world? No man is an island, entire of itself; every man is a piece of the continent, a part of the main. If a clod be washed away by the sea, Europe is the less, as well as if a promontory were, as well as if a manor of thy friend's or of thine own were; any man's death diminishes me, because I am involved in mankind; and therefore never send to know

for whom the bell tolls; it tolls for thee." J. Donne, Meditation No. 17, Devotions Upon Emergent Occasions 86, 87 (A. Raspa ed. 1987).

9. See 497 U.S., at 332, n. 2.

10. "[N]either the Bill of Rights nor the laws of sovereign States create the liberty which the Due Process Clause protects. The relevant constitutional provisions are limitations on the power of the sovereign to infringe on the liberty of the citizen. The relevant state laws either create property rights, or they curtail the freedom of the citizen who must live in an ordered society. Of course, law is essential to the exercise and enjoyment of individual liberty in a complex society. But it is not the source of liberty, and surely not the exclusive source.

"I had thought it self evident that all men were endowed by their Creator with liberty as one of the cardinal unalienable rights. It is that basic freedom which the Due Process Clause protects, rather than the particular rights or privileges conferred by specific laws or regulations." *Meachum* v. *Fano*, 427 U.S. 215, 230 (1976) (Stevens, J., dissenting).

11. "Nancy Cruzan's interest in life, no less than that of any other person, includes an interest in how she will be thought of after her death by those whose opinions mattered to her. There can be no doubt that her life made her dear to her family and to others. How she dies will affect how that life is remembered." *Cruzan* v. *Director, Mo. Dept. of Health*, 497 U.S. 261, 344 (1990) (Stevens, J., dissenting).

"Each of us has an interest in the kind of memories that will survive after death. To that end, individual decisions are often motivated by their impact on others. A member of the kind of family identified in the trial court's findings in this case would likely have not only a normal interest in minimizing the burden that her own illness imposes on others, but also an interest in having their memories of her filled predominantly with thoughts about her past vitality rather than her current condition." *Id.,* at 356.

12. I note that there is evidence that a significant number of physicians support the practice of hastening death in particular situations. A survey published in the New England Journal of Medicine, found that 56% of responding doctors in Michigan preferred legalizing assisted suicide to an explicit ban. Bachman et al., Attitudes of Michigan Physicians and the Public Toward Legalizing Physician Assisted Suicide and Voluntary Euthanasia, 334 New England J. Med. 303-309 (1996). In a survey of Oregon doctors, 60% of the responding doctors supported legalizing assisted suicide for terminally ill patients. See Lee et al., Legalizing Assisted Suicide—Views of Physicians in Oregon, 335 New England J. Med. 310-315 (1996). Another study showed that 12% of physicians polled in Washington State reported that they had been asked by their terminally ill patients for prescriptions to hasten death, and that, in the year prior to the study, 24% of those physicians had complied with such requests. See Back, Wallace, Starks, & Perlman, Physician Assisted Suicide and Euthanasia in Washington State, 275 JAMA 919-925 (1996); see also Doukas, Waterhouse, Gorenflo, & Seld, Attitudes and Behaviors on Physician Assisted Death: A Study of Michigan Oncologists, 13 J. Clinical Oncology 1055 (1995) (reporting

that 18% of responding Michigan oncologists reported active participation in assisted suicide); Slome, Moulton, Huffine, Gorter, & Abrams, Physicians' Attitudes Toward Assisted Suicide in AIDS, 5 J. Acquired Immune Deficiency Syndromes 712 (1992) (reporting that 24% of responding physicians who treat AIDS patients would likely grant a patient's request for assistance in hastening death).

13. See *Vacco* v. *Quill, ante,* at 1, nn. 1 and 2.

14. The American Medical Association recognized this distinction when it supported Nancy Cruzan and continues to recognize this distinction in its support of the States in these cases.

15. If a doctor prescribes lethal drugs to be self administered by the patient, it not at all clear that the physician's intent is that the patient "be made dead," *ante,* at 7 (internal quotation marks omitted). Many patients prescribed lethal medications never actually take them; they merely acquire some sense of control in the process of dying that the availability of those medications provides. See Back, *supra* n. 12, at 922; see also Quill, 324 New England J. Med., at 693 (describing how some patients fear death less when they feel they have the option of physician assisted suicide).

Supreme Court of the United States

DENNIS C. VACCO, ATTORNEY GENERAL OF NEW YORK, ET AL., PETITIONERS 95-1858 *v.* TIMOTHY E. QUILL ET AL.

On Writ of Certiorari to the United States Court of Appeals for the Second Circuit

[JUNE 26, 1997]

Justice Souter, concurring in the judgment.

Even though I do not conclude that assisted suicide is a fundamental right entitled to recognition at this time, I accord the claims raised by the patients and physicians in this case and *Washington* v. *Glucksberg* a high degree of importance, requiring a commensurate justification. See *Washington* v. *Glucksberg, ante,* at 24-41 (Souter, J., concurring in judgment). The reasons that lead me to conclude in *Glucksberg* that the prohibition on assisted suicide is not arbitrary under the due process standard also support the distinction between assistance to suicide, which is banned, and practices such as termination of artificial life support and death hastening pain medication, which are permitted. I accordingly concur in the judgment of the Court.

Supreme Court of the United States

WASHINGTON ET AL., PETITIONERS 96-110 *v.* HAROLD
GLUCKSBERG ET AL.

ON WRIT OF CERTIORARI TO THE UNITED STATES COURT OF APPEALS
FOR THE NINTH CIRCUIT

DENNIS C. VACCO, ATTORNEY GENERAL OF NEW YORK, ET
AL., PETITIONERS 95-1858 *v.* TIMOTHY E. QUILL ET AL.

ON WRIT OF CERTIORARI TO THE UNITED STATES COURT OF APPEALS
FOR THE SECOND CIRCUIT

[JUNE 26, 1997]

Justice Ginsburg, concurring in the judgments.

I concur in the Court's judgments in these cases substantially for the reasons
stated by Justice O'Connor in her concurring opinion.

Supreme Court of the United States

WASHINGTON ET AL., PETITIONERS 96-110 *v.* HAROLD
GLUCKSBERG ET AL.

ON WRIT OF CERTIORARI TO THE UNITED STATES COURT OF APPEALS
FOR THE NINTH CIRCUIT

DENNIS C. VACCO, ATTORNEY GENERAL OF NEW YORK, ET
AL., PETITIONERS 95-1858 *v.* TIMOTHY E. QUILL ET AL.

ON WRIT OF CERTIORARI TO THE UNITED STATES COURT OF APPEALS
FOR THE SECOND CIRCUIT

[JUNE 26, 1997]

Justice Breyer, concurring in the judgments.

I believe that Justice O'Connor's views, which I share, have greater legal
significance than the Court's opinion suggests. I join her separate opinion,
except insofar as it joins the majority. And I concur in the judgments. I shall
briefly explain how I differ from the Court.

I agree with the Court in *Vacco* v. *Quill, ante,* that the articulated state interests justify the distinction drawn between physician assisted suicide and withdrawal of life support. I also agree with the Court that the critical question in
both of the cases before us is whether "the 'liberty' specially protected by the
Due Process Clause includes a right" of the sort that the respondents assert.
Washington v. *Glucksberg, ante,* at 19. I do not agree, however, with the Court's
formulation of that claimed "liberty" interest. The Court describes it as a "right
to commit suicide with another's assistance." *Ante,* at 20. But I would not reject
the respondents' claim without considering a different formulation, for which
our legal tradition may provide greater support. That formulation would use
words roughly like a "right to die with dignity." But irrespective of the exact
words used, at its core would lie personal control over the manner of death,
professional medical assistance, and the avoidance of unnecessary and severe
physical suffering—combined.

As Justice Souter points out, *ante* at 13-16 (Souter, J., concurring in the
judgment), Justice Harlan's dissenting opinion in *Poe* v. *Ullman,* 367 U.S. 497
(1961), offers some support for such a claim. In that opinion, Justice Harlan
referred to the "liberty" that the Fourteenth Amendment protects as including "a freedom from all substantial arbitrary impositions and purposeless restraints" and also as recognizing that "*certain interests* require particularly careful scrutiny of the state needs asserted to justify their abridgment." *Id.,* at 543.
The "certain interests" to which Justice Harlan referred may well be similar
(perhaps identical) to the rights, liberties, or interests that the Court today, as
in the past, regards as "fundamental." *Ante,* at 15; see also *Planned Parenthood
of Southeastern Pa.* v. *Casey,* 505 U.S. 833 (1992); *Eisenstadt* v. *Baird,* 405 U.S.
438 (1972); *Griswold* v. *Connecticut,* 381 U.S. 479 (1965); *Rochin* v. *California,*
342 U.S. 165 (1952); *Skinner* v. *Oklahoma ex rel. Williamson,* 316 U.S. 535 (1942).

Justice Harlan concluded that marital privacy was such a "special interest."
He found in the Constitution a right of "privacy of the home"—with the home,
the bedroom, and "intimate details of the marital relation" at its heart—by
examining the protection that the law had earlier provided for related, but not
identical, interests described by such words as "privacy," "home," and "family."
367 U.S., at 548, 552; cf. *Casey, supra,* at 851. The respondents here essentially
ask us to do the same. They argue that one can find a "right to die with dignity"
by examining the protection the law has provided for related, but not identical,
interests relating to personal dignity, medical treatment, and freedom from
state inflicted pain. See *Ingraham* v. *Wright,* 430 U.S. 651 (1977); *Cruzan* v.
Director, Mo. Dept. of Health, 497 U.S. 261 (1990); *Casey, supra.*

I do not believe, however, that this Court need or now should decide
whether or a not such a right is "fundamental." That is because, in my view,
the avoidance of severe physical pain (connected with death) would have to
comprise an essential part of any successful claim and because, as Justice
O'Connor points out, the laws before us do not *force* a dying person to undergo
that kind of pain. *Ante,* at 2 (O'Connor, J., concurring). Rather, the laws of
New York and of Washington do not prohibit doctors from providing patients
with drugs sufficient to control pain despite the risk that those drugs themselves will kill. Cf. New York State Task Force on Life and the Law, When Death

Is Sought: Assisted Suicide and Euthanasia in the Medical Context 163, n. 29 (May 1994). And under these circumstances the laws of New York and Washington would overcome any remaining significant interests and would be justified, regardless.

Medical technology, we are repeatedly told, makes the administration of pain relieving drugs sufficient, except for a very few individuals for whom the ineffectiveness of pain control medicines can mean, not pain, but the need for sedation which can end in a coma. Brief for National Hospice Organization 8; Brief for the American Medical Association (AMA) et al. as *Amici Curiae* 6; see also Byock, Consciously Walking the Fine Line: Thoughts on a Hospice Response to Assisted Suicide and Euthanasia, 9 J. Palliative Care 25, 26 (1993); New York State Task Force, at 44, and n. 37. We are also told that there are many instances in which patients do not receive the palliative care that, in principle, is available, *id.,* at 43-47; Brief for AMA as *Amici Curiae* 6; Brief for Choice in Dying, Inc., as *Amici Curiae* 20, but that is so for institutional reasons or inadequacies or obstacles, which would seem possible to overcome, and which do *not* include *a prohibitive set of laws. Ante,* at 2 (O'Connor, J., concurring); see also 2 House of Lords, Session 1993-1994 Report of Select Committee on Medical Ethics 113 (1994) (indicating that the number of palliative care centers in the United Kingdom, where physician assisted suicide is illegal, significantly exceeds that in the Netherlands, where such practices are legal).

This legal circumstance means that the state laws before us do not infringe directly upon the (assumed) central interest (what I have called the core of the interest in dying with dignity) as, by way of contrast, the state anticontraceptive laws at issue in *Poe* did interfere with the central interest there at stake—by bringing the State's police powers to bear upon the marital bedroom.

Were the legal circumstances different—for example, were state law to prevent the provision of palliative care, including the administration of drugs as needed to avoid pain at the end of life—then the law's impact upon serious and otherwise unavoidable physical pain (accompanying death) would be more directly at issue. And as Justice O'Connor suggests, the Court might have to revisit its conclusions in these cases.

CONTRIBUTORS

ARTHUR L. CAPLAN, Ph.D., is director of the Center for Bioethics and Trustee Professor at the University of Pennsylvania. He is the author or editor of more than 25 books and nearly 600 articles in journals of medicine, philosophy, and biology.

THE REVEREND RALPH CIAMPA, S.T.M., is director of the Department of Pastoral Care at the University of Pennsylvania Health System and a member of the Hospital of the University of Pennsylvania Institutional Ethics Committee. A United Methodist minister and chaplain, he oversees an interfaith program of patient care, clinical pastoral education, spirituality, health research, and community partnerships.

BARBARA COOMBS LEE, P.A., F.N.P., J.D., is president of Compassion in Dying, an organization to improve end-of-life care and expand choices. Educated at Vassar College, Cornell University, the University of Washington, and Lewis and Clark Law School, she has practiced as a nurse practitioner, physician assistant, and attorney. Her publications address health care, law, and policy.

FRANK DAVIDOFF, M.D., is editor of the *Annals of Internal Medicine*. He received his medical degree from Columbia University and has held academic appointments at Harvard Medical School and the University of Connecticut School of Medicine. He was formerly senior vice-president for education at the American College of Physicians and has published extensively on clinical medicine and health policy issues.

KATHY FABER-LANGENDOEN, M.D., is director of the State University of New York (SUNY) Upstate Medical University's Center for Bioethics and Humanities as well as a practicing oncologist. Her research focuses on ethical issues in the care of patients dying in intensive care units.

JOSEPH J. FINS, M.D., is director of medical ethics, associate professor of medicine, and associate professor of medicine in psychiatry at New York Presbyterian Hospital and Cornell's Weill Medical College. He is a recipient of a Project on Death in America Faculty Scholars Award and a Woodrow Wilson Visiting Fellowship, and he served on the White House Commission on Complementary and Alternative Medicine Policy during the Clinton administration.

KATRINA HEDBERG, M.D., M.P.H., is the deputy state epidemiologist for the Oregon Health Division, Department of Human Services. She oversees the mandated reporting system for Oregon's Death with Dignity Act, which legalizes physician-assisted suicide for terminally ill Oregon residents. She has co-authored articles on Oregon's experience with physician-assisted suicide that were published in the *New England Journal of Medicine.*

JASON H. T. KARLAWISH, M.D., is an assistant professor in the Department of Medicine and a fellow of the Center for Bioethics at the University of Pennsylvania. He is associate director of the Memory Disorders Clinic and directs the Alzheimer's Disease Center's Education and Information Transfer Core. His awards include a Brookdale National Fellowship, a Paul Beeson Fellowship, and *Lancet's* Wakley prize.

FRANKLIN G. MILLER, Ph.D., is special expert, National Institute of Mental Health Intramural Research Program and Department of Clinical Bioethics, National Institutes of Health. Previously, he taught bioethics at the University of Virginia. Miller has published on the ethics of clinical research, death and dying, professional integrity, and pragmatism and bioethics.

SALLY J. NUNN, R.N., is a fellow and director of clinical outreach at the University of Pennsylvania Center for Bioethics. She does bioethics consulting and directs the Ethics Network of the Delaware Valley Region. She cofounded and was long-time director of the Southern Jersey Ethics Alliance, a consortium of fifty-one health care institutions.

DAVID ORENTLICHER, M.D., J.D., is Samuel R. Rosen Professor at Indiana University School of Law, Indianapolis. He also has an adjunct appointment in medicine at the Indiana University School of Medicine. He is the author of a forthcoming book, *Matters of Life and Death.* He graduated from Harvard Medical School and Harvard Law School.

PETER POON, J.D., M.A., oversees the Department of Veterans Affairs research misconduct program, Office of Research Compliance and Assurance. He has practiced law and worked in the field of bioethics, and he holds degrees in bioethics from Brown University and the University of Washington and in law from the University of California, Berkeley.

TIMOTHY E. QUILL, M.D., is professor of medicine, psychiatry, and medical humanities at the University of Rochester School of Medicine and Dentistry and a primary care internist. He is a graduate of Amherst College and the University of Rochester. His most recent book is *A Midwife through the Dying Process: Stories of Healing and Hard Choices at the End of Life* (1996).

ELLIOTT J. ROSEN, Ed.D., is director of the Family Institute of Westchester in White Plains, New York, and consulting psychologist with Phelps Memorial Hospice in Sleepy Hollow, New York. He directs the behavioral science curriculum in the Mercy College Graduate Physician Assistant program and serves on the Ethics Committee of the National Hospice and Palliative Care Organization.

LOIS SNYDER, J.D., is adjunct assistant professor of bioethics and fellow of the University of Pennsylvania Center for Bioethics. She also directs the Center for Ethics and Professionalism at the American College of Physicians-American Society of Internal Medicine. A graduate of the University of Pennsylvania and Temple University School of Law, she frequently writes and speaks on health policy, bioethical, and medical-legal issues. Her most recent book is *Physician's Guide to End-of-Life Care* (2001).

SUSAN W. TOLLE, M.D., is a practicing internist and serves as director of the multidisciplinary Center for Ethics in Health Care at Oregon Health Sciences University. Tolle and the Center for Ethics in Health Care remain neutral on the issue of physician-assisted suicide and have instead focused energies on improving the humane care of the terminally ill.

JAMES A. TULSKY, M.D., is director of the Program on the Medical Encounter and Palliative Care at the Durham (North Carolina) VA Medical Center. He is also associate professor of medicine and associate director of the Institute on Care at the End of Life at Duke University.

Note: Affiliations are for identification only.

INDEX